DATE DUE

DEMCO 38-296

In a Tangled Wood

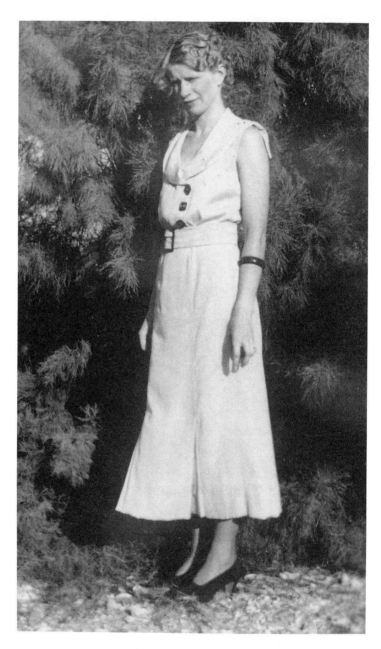

Annabelle Haberkost, ca. 1935

In a Tangled Wood

An Alzheimer's Journey

JOYCE DYER

FOREWORD BY IAN FRAZIER

Southern Methodist University Press
Dallas

First edition, 1996

Copyright acknowledgments appear on pages 159–60.

Requests for permission to reproduce material from this work
should be sent to:
Permissions
Southern Methodist University Press
PO Box 750415
Dallas, TX 75275-0415

Library of Congress Cataloging-in-Publication Data
Dyer, Joyce.
    In a tangled wood : an Alzheimer's journey / Joyce Dyer :
foreword by Ian Frazier. — 1st. ed.
        p.   cm.
    Includes bibliographical references.
    ISBN 0-87074-396-1 (cloth). — ISBN 0-87074-397-X (paper)
    1. Coyne, Edna Annabelle Haberkost—Health. 2. Alzheimer's
disease—Popular works. 3. Alzheimer's disease—Patients—Family
relationships. 4. Alzheimer's disease—Patients—Nursing home care.
I. Title.
RC523.2.D94   1994
362.1'96831'0092—dc20
    [B]   96-11354

Text design by Barbara Whitehead
Cover design by Tom Dawson Graphic Design

Printed in the United States of America on acid-free paper
10   9   8   7   6   5   4   3   2   1

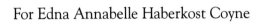
For Edna Annabelle Haberkost Coyne

tanglewood, n. A region of thick, bushy woods.
1853 N. HAWTHORNE (*title*), Tanglewood
Tales, for Girls and Boys. 1863 MITCHELL.
My Farm 158 Within this tangle-wood, I have
set a few graftlings upon a wild-crab.
1894 *Advance* 26 April, [The bird] scuttled
off in a wild panic through the thick tanglewood.

A *Dictionary of Americanisms*
on Historical Principles

∿

And I—like one lost in a thorny wood
That rents the thorns and is rent with the thorns,
Seeking a way and straying from the way;
Not knowing how to find the open air,
But toiling desperately to find it out—
Torment myself. . . .

SHAKESPEARE,
King Henry the Sixth—Part Three

Contents

FOREWORD

All that Alzheimer's disease takes away—independence, identity, memory, and finally life—reveals itself as precious in slow motion as it disappears. To love a person who has the disease is to suffer each loss in turn, making up each deficit the best you can. Independence had kept the rules between the two of you, but as the person with the disease loses all of hers, you give up much of yours to care for her and be with her. When her identity begins to fade, you realize that your own is attached to it, and you shore hers up as if in self-defense, with new clothes and hair styles and the right words in her mouth when her conversation fails. Most of all, what was shared between you required memory, and in larger and larger amounts you must borrow from your own to fill the supply. At first you provide a name or a date or a detail when it won't come; later you add whole paragraphs; finally, everything that is to be remembered relies only on you. It is this last and strongest imperative that drives *In a Tangled Wood: An Alzheimer's Journey*, Joyce Dyer's loving and hard-won retrieval of her mother. In defiance of the disease, Ms. Dyer vowed not to forget a single thing.

As the person who is sick forgets who you are, you sometimes forget what she was like before the disease. New, hard-to-erase images intervene, images of disintegration and helplessness and confusion, lit sometimes by words and acts that would have mortified her, before. An offhand trick of the disease, but a cruel one, is to leave this memory freshest in the minds of those who survive. Afterwards, you may be compelled to crack the glaze of those images, to break through to memories of the person as she used to be. Grief may make a historian of you, an archaeologist of the ordinary details that evoke the vanished person's life. You become, usually too late, a biographer. Through recollection, Ms. Dyer is these and more. The simple fact that her mother served in the Food Service division of the Akron, Ohio, public schools from 1928 to 1973, and that she loved her job, takes on the strength of a paradigm when set among the author's observations of the gentle institution where her mother's life will end. Another author might have chosen to fast-forward through the inevitabilities of this endgame. Ms. Dyer chooses instead to look hard at each living moment of her mother's decline, to find unexpected revelation there.

Photographs of what Alzheimer's does to a brain would not lead you to suspect how much of a sufferer's personality remains throughout. By watching with patient affection, Ms. Dyer catches these flashes of essential self as they appear among the apparently random or chaotic behavior not only of her mother but of the other patients in the ward. An Alzheimer's personality becomes a riddle expressed in ever more far-flung or inscrutable terms. And yet at those brief moments of connection when the riddle is solved, the true soul shines through all the brighter for the difficulties involved. With her devotion as credentials, Ms. Dyer fits in easily among the nurses and therapists who work at Tanglewood, joining them in an understanding of the place's unique reality. Because she understands, she is one of them, and can portray them convincingly as the near-saints they often are. The reader comes to share Ms. Dyer's gratitude to these men and women who know about the disease and can dispel part of its fearfulness.

An Alzheimer's ward is full of imaginary people: near each patient, a step behind or off to one side, is the suggestion of the person he or she used to be. The best of those who care for the sick at Tanglewood seem to keep both the real and the imaginary—the present sufferer, and that sufferer's former self—simultaneously in mind. If you are, as Ms. Dyer was, not an employee but a daily visitor to the ward, and if like her you are visiting a parent, the parent's former self is your regular companion. Perhaps you even have silent conversations with this person you recall so clearly. You can imagine her, in some ideal afterworld with all slates clean and all illness cured, laughing at the wild things she's doing now. You accept each momentary reality of the person you love as you would the stages of a child; each stage is just a sketch, an aspect of the whole personality, and worthy to be loved. The unqualified nature of Ms. Dyer's acceptance of her mother gives her observations not only unity but a certain transcendent calm.

If some of the imaginary people in the ward are from the past, some also are from the future. The doctors and therapists and nurses, most of them younger than most of the patients, will of course one day be old themselves. This disease could be waiting for them. We sense in the attention they give their patients an awareness that the disease has a claim not only on its current victims but on the rest of us as well. As Ms. Dyer notes, children of Alzheimer's victims are more likely than others to get the disease. Lying underneath her narrative, this threat adds a poignancy to it: like all of us who have witnessed a parent's destruction by Alzheimer's, she knows she could be looking at a future version of herself.

When my father had Alzheimer's, I worried constantly that my own memory was starting to go. The least slip of the mind could send me into fits of self-examination to see if the brain was still on line. Once on a long train ride I found myself unable to recall the name of former Notre Dame football coach Ara Parseghian. Ara Parseghian is a euphonious name, and pleasant on the tongue, but that was all I could remember of it. I couldn't get to a telephone or a reference book, and I spent hours throwing mental filing cabinets around looking for the name Ara Parseghian. These minor episodes, when I was in the middle of them, seemed to go on and on. I imagined this was how my father had often felt in the early stages of the disease. As his illness progressed into its fifth year, I told my uncle that I thought it would never end. He said, "Oh, it will." Just that small amount of assurance gave me comfort. When you're close to the disease you don't know that it will end, or that it has any form or reason or sense to it at all. You know that it is pain, and that it changes but generally and inexorably gets worse—and not much more. Then you learn that it does in fact end, and as you move farther from it in time you see that it had a structure both specific and general, like other acts of nature. You see that there's no lesson of Alzheimer's, no moral or meaning you could sum up in a sentence. But there is a certain integrity to the way it all played out, a fitness you can feel but not touch with any words short of the accumulating words of narrative.

When I cast my own family's experience of Alzheimer's as a narrative, I stopped worrying about forgetting things. In fact, I believe that not only did I stop worrying about forgetting, I actually stopped forgetting things as well. Narrative heals. A narrative assembled with the attentiveness Ms. Dyer has given to hers knits and makes stronger the places that were weak, not only for herself and her family but for the reader too. Meaning, though woven throughout her narrative, is difficult to pull from it in a single strand. Meaning is not only in the story she tells but in the book itself, in the physical object you hold in your hand. Having myself written a book from similar experience, I can say that no other response to the disease seemed as apt. A book defies the chaos and nothingness of Alzheimer's; it stands up to it and takes down names and answers back. When my father was sick I liked to read the Ezra Pound poem with the line, "What thou lovest well remains." Ms. Dyer shows us that what remains is an immense survival, despite the worst the disease can do. Her book is a marker, a reply, and an act of the special boldness one is granted by love.

Ian Frazier

PREFACE

My mother, Edna Annabelle Haberkost Coyne, was diagnosed with Alzheimer's disease in 1986. As her illness grew progressively worse, it became impossible for me to care for her alone. The middle and late stages of Alzheimer's affect far more than memory. There were behavior changes caused by Annabelle Coyne's poor decaying brain that made her dangerous to herself, dangerous, at times, to others.

The decision to find a "home" for my mother was perhaps the most painful decision of my life. I remembered only my visits as a girl to the nursing home where my Grandmother Coyne spent her last years. She was diagnosed back in the late '50s with "hardening of the arteries," but it was probably Alzheimer's disease, now that I think about it. The "home" Bessie Coyne was in consisted of a ward of steel hospital beds. When we visited my grandmother on Sunday afternoons, she was always heavily sedated and always lying on her back. No one at the home ever spoke to her. It was a horrible place.

I'm afraid such places still exist. But Tanglewood is not one of them. Something, nothing less than a miracle and sheer luck, led me to its doors when I desperately needed help in the late summer of 1990. The summer when I knew that neither my mother nor I could survive this disease much longer by ourselves.

I am supremely thankful that my mother was not born any earlier than she was. Beginning in the late '80s, kind and competent individuals everywhere were starting to understand that people with Alzheimer's needed a unique environment, and if that environment could be created, they would be able to function far better, far more happily than in a traditional home setting. Professionals would begin insisting, among other things, that "patients" in Alzheimer-specific units be called "residents."

This book takes you inside an Alzheimer's unit. Tanglewood is the name I've given this unit, but it represents life inside many such units. During the course of Annabelle's illness, she resided primarily in one wonderful center, but not one exclusively. I visited numerous Alzheimer's units during her illness and nearly always was moved by what I saw. Tanglewood represents them all—those that I visited, those where my mother lived.

In many ways, the sick and their families must walk through this disease alone. And yet, places like Tanglewood make every step of that inevitable journey less frightening. Mysteriously, and beyond all understanding, Tanglewood drew me in. I felt at home there. I learned to love its residents and soon found myself living by the rhythms and cycles of my mother's institution.

Tanglewood is a community of people who understand AD in all its strangeness and horror. Residents are freer there than they could be anywhere else in the world. Acceptance of the most bizarre behavior imaginable is complete and absolute. Tenderness accompanies even the most ordinary act. Dignity still remains after residents don diapers and have in their mouths neither teeth nor words. At Tanglewood, all that can be done for the disease *is* done.

The names of residents, other than my mother, are not real. I have changed them to protect privacy, to protect the astonishing innocence of my friends. Some details have also occasionally been altered for the same purpose, as well as for the sake of compression and structure. Composite characters walk onto the pages now and then.

Most of the segments in these chapters occurred during the summer of 1994, though some took place much earlier, and a few much later. Flashbacks will help you understand the progression of my mother's disease, as well as the extent and nature of her valor.

Many communities have helped support me throughout the

years of my mother's illness. In the selected annotated bibliography you will find at the end, as well as in my epigraphs to chapters, I try to identify and thank one in particular: the community of writers struggling to understand not only changes in the brains of people with AD but also changes in ourselves that necessarily accompany such devastating alterations in those close to us. Alzheimer's no longer is the closeted disease it once was. The literature of Alzheimer's is growing, and with that growth has come better understanding.

This book attempts to help relatives of those seriously ill with Alzheimer's recognize that profoundly new concepts in the management and care of this incurable disease are working and should be explored—without guilt or sorrow. There are now four million Americans stricken with Alzheimer's. But there are an additional nineteen million caring for them. A total of twenty-three million Americans, in other words, suffer from Alzheimer's in this country and need comprehensive help.

Caregivers trying to locate Alzheimer's units should begin by contacting the National Alzheimer's Association (919 N. Michigan Avenue, Suite 1000, Chicago, IL 60611, 1-800-272-3900 or 312-335-8700). The National Association will know which of its over a thousand chapters is closest to individual caregivers and will provide this information. Most local chapters will mail family members a list of area facilities for those suffering from Alzheimer's. Such listings usually specify whether a nursing home offers an Alzheimer's unit, an Alzheimer's specialty, or an Alzheimer's program.

The National Institute on Aging supplies even more specific information on special care units. The Alzheimer's Disease Education and Referral Center (ADEAR) at the National Institute on Aging (1-800-438-4380) can provide referral phone numbers closer to people's homes. Caregivers receive nursing home profiles, including number of beds, average age of residents, Medicare and Medicaid status, waiting period for admission, and special medical programs available.

But this is not enough. Even after information has been gathered from the Alzheimer's Association and the Institute on Aging, it's essential to visit units and spend time in them, watching and listening.

I hope that reading about Tanglewood will help those who are now standing where I was only a few short years ago see institutions with clearer eyes. I found Tanglewood by luck. But there are better ways. I hope my book will let others know when they have arrived where they need to be.

My book also has one or two other ambitions. I try to explain how the disease charts its course by looking at residents who are in every stage of the illness. I try not to shy away from later stages, believing that knowing what is ahead sometimes makes it easier to prepare ourselves to watch. And I try to assure my readers that although Alzheimer's is devastating and tragic, it also, inexplicably, brings moments of grace and joy and understanding.

Perhaps more than anything, my book attempts to convey my love for the guardian angels at Tanglewood, for its amazing residents, and, most of all, for Edna Annabelle Haberkost Coyne.

Joyce Dyer

ACKNOWLEDGMENTS

I once thought there was great virtue in doing difficult things alone. Alzheimer's disease showed me how wrong I was. My book is an acknowledgment of the absolute importance of community to get through times like these, an acknowledgment of the generosity of the human spirit. There is not room to list the names of everyone who stayed close to me during the nine years of my mother's illness. They know I will hold them, always, in memory. But I cannot leave this page without thanking a few special people and organizations who have treated me, and my book, with unusual affection and attentiveness.

And so I thank Dr. Marty Klipec, Cindy Brodsky, Anne-Marie Gustavson, Jane McAvoy, Roger Adkins, and Nancy Rosenberg—my early readers who cheered me on and offered excellent suggestions. I thank, especially, my dear colleague Carol Donley, director of the Center for Literature, Medicine, and the Health Care Professions at Hiram College, for her boundless encouragement and assistance. I thank Jerry Brodsky for his quiet strength, and quiet tears, and Pat and Bill Eldredge for taking me into their home on a lonely Christmas Eve. I thank Richard Dyer, Dave Dyer, Janice McCormick, Ronald and Nola Osborn, and Ed Dyer for their love and concern. And friends like Sandra Parker, for always sensing when I needed help—and providing it. I thank the nurses, doctors, staff members, administrators, and residents who loved my mother exactly as she was.

I am immensely grateful to Dr. Peter J. Whitehouse, professor of neurology and director of the University Hospitals of Cleveland Alzheimer Center. One of our country's most talented people in the area of Alzheimer's research, diagnosis, and treatment, he still found time to serve as medical consultant to my book. His comments were invaluable to me.

I could not have made the progress I was able to on my book during the summer of 1994 without the vigorous assistance of Tom Vince and his library staff at the Hudson Library and Historical Society, and without Lisa Johnson, Mary Lou Selander, Pat Basu, Jeff Wanser, Erma Fritsche, and other library staff at Hiram College. I thank Millie Schwan for her unfailing interest in this project and her professional assistance. I thank Hiram College faculty, staff, and administrators for their unexpected response to an early reading from *In a Tangled Wood*. And I thank Hiram College for its support of my work through generous awards from the Gerstacker-Gund Summer Fellowship Fund and the Michael Dively Endowment for Scholarly Publications.

I'll always be grateful to Wendell and Marie Scott, to Isabelle Crutchfield and her daughter Patricia, to Prudence Dyer, and to Paul and Edith Steurer for visiting my mother. I lovingly thank my son, Stephen Osborn Dyer, for his valiant attempts to enter Annabelle's world. And there is no way to explain what it meant to have a husband who for five years prepared my meals and did everything else that needed to be done, without complaint, without any desire for notice or thanks, so that I could care for Annabelle Coyne. There is no question in my mind that Daniel Osborn Dyer kept me alive through this difficult time.

Finally, in memory, I thank my parents. I am the only daughter, the only child, of Thomas and Annabelle Coyne, born to them when they were nearly forty years old. They had very little, worked harder than any two people I've ever known, and loved me with their dying breath. They taught me that it's not good to let your heart be broken by little things. A heart must be made of very sturdy stuff to get through this life. They taught me how to be happy, and how to survive. They gave me leisure when I was young, something they never had. And I like to think that in that gift they gave me time to learn the craft that would one day be used to tell their story.

In a Tangled Wood

A large sign engraved with the words *The Woods Center for the Aging* greets visitors at the entrance by the road. The sign is white, stenciled on every edge with a border of pines. In the middle are listed the levels of care provided inside the brick building at the end of the long drive.

Independent Living
Assisted Living
Nursing

But there is no mention of Tanglewood, the Alzheimer's unit housed in the far west corner of the complex.

You have trouble locating Tanglewood even after you enter the main building. There are no arrows to direct you. You must find your own way, blindly winding through a maze of narrow halls.

When you reach the end of the nursing wing, a pair of heavy steel doors suddenly confronts you. On them are two long panes of pale amber glass, reinforced with thin wire, and a small sign: *Press Red Button on Wall Before Entering*. You have arrived.

As ominous as the doors are, they attract you. You want to open them and see what they hide. The panels of reinforced glass are draped on the inside with ancient lace. You want to touch it. Tanglewood houses twenty-four Alzheimer's residents and was added on to The Woods only five years ago. Perhaps that explains why the sign at the lip of the road is out of date.

Or maybe Tanglewood isn't mentioned because the idea that our minds will vanish from our heads, that our brain cells will dry up like fall leaves and blow away one night in the middle of our sleep, is something too horrible to think about. Something best not announced on a public street.

Tanglewood is on the outskirts of town. It is a very private world. Those who go there to live do not return. And those who visit are never the same again.

CHAPTER ONE

Family

NARRATOR: . . . *Tomorrow or next month, I will be somebody else. Ruth, Bernice, Elaine, who knows. Someday she will call me mother because her mother will be all she remembers.*

JO CARSON, *Daytrips*

·1·

In the hall across from us, I see a new resident sitting in a chair. She is better dressed and more vocal than others here. A woman passes her, and smiles. The new resident, dressed in green, with bright henna hair, has something to say. "Every player has to make money, honey," she shouts. "Wave your magic wand, and everything will happen."

"I don't have a wand," the woman passing by stutters, confused, grabbing the loose flesh on her neck with her left hand.

"Yes you do," the new resident winks. "You're carrying one."

She nods toward the floor. The woman with turkey flesh discovers her cane in her right hand and gleefully passes it through the air over the head of the emerald queen.

·2·

"You!" the woman in green shouts my way. "Come here. I need to talk to you." I check my mother, see that she's all right, and walk just a few steps to meet the woman in polyester green. "I'm Gloria Nevel," she instructs me, staring through filmy green eyes. "I'm George's aunt. Tell them I send lots of love. Lots. You hear me? LOTS."

"I will, Gloria," I smile, taking her hand and starting to turn away.

"Wait!" she orders. "Do you play the piano?" Gloria points in the direction of the spinet that church groups use when they conduct services in Tanglewood.

"No," I tell her.

"Too bad," Gloria says. "I thought you could play and drive them all out of here. Get rid of 'em for me. I need some sleep."

·3·

Angie, the activity director, has guided the others outdoors. They are batting a pink beach ball in the air, when they remember how.

My mother has not joined them. She is squeezing chair seats when I arrive, testing them, looking for the softest one. She can choose the most comfortable seat in the house today. She's in the La-Z-Boy showroom on Main Street, all by herself.

The others return about 4:00 P.M. from their exercise. Kathleen McGraw is laughing, walking more briskly than usual, teasing a ten-year-old boy who volunteers in Tanglewood during the summer. She sits beside me. The boy sits to her left.

"We had this boy with us today," she whispers in my ear. "We tried to make him feel important."

The TV is on in the background, though the sound is off. Kathleen glances toward it. "I can remember when TV was a brand new thing. We thought it was a miracle. It *is*, if you stop to think about it."

"It's 'getting-to-know-you' time before dinner!" Angie announces. "We're going to find out about our families."

"'Getting to Know You'!" Kathleen breaks into song. Her voice is clear and powerful.

The refreshment cart screeches in, with a plump aide at the wheel. For the next ten minutes the director is upstaged by diet Shasta ginger ale, pineapple and cranberry juice, lemonade, Snapple.

"I wonder if she keeps coffee on that thing?" Kathleen asks me, warm coffee from her past still streaming in her veins.

The activity director begins with Helen. "How many brothers and sisters did you have, Helen?" she asks.

My mother has gone to sleep, along with the blue parakeet and the canary in the cage to our left.

"I had a very good life," Helen begins. "There were five of us. Frieda was my favorite. She was the oldest and handed out the advice."

Kathleen hears the noise of dinner preparation beginning in the background. "I hope whoever's in the kitchen isn't tearing it apart!" she laughs, then yawns, uninterested in Helen's answers. "I'm hungry."

"And you, Mr. Miller? How many siblings?"

"Four brothers," he says curtly, tipping his Miller Dairy baseball cap in her direction. "I was the baby. We harvested crops together and got along. Grew corn, wheat, oats, rye."

Beautiful Mrs. Blackburn is dreaming and waiting to tell her tale. Helen acts as her coach, her agent, her most loyal fan.

"I was born in New York City," says Mrs. Blackburn in a thick accent that verifies her claim.

"Bet that was nice," Helen interrupts. "A lot of active stuff going on?"

"My parents owned a confectioner's shop," Mrs. Blackburn continues, adjusting the fur piece that wraps her shoulders.

"And she comes from an interesting place," Helen again interrupts.

"In Manhattan. The big bridge opened. The Brooklyn Bridge. My parents and my brother and I lived above the store."

Mrs. Blackburn's memory swims with her mother's, with her grandmother's, as she recalls the opening of the Brooklyn Bridge in 1883.

"And your brother?" Angie inquires.

"My brother went to a big place to take his piano lessons. That's our piano!" Mrs. Blackburn points to the spinet in the room. "We had forty or fifty tables and chairs and a piano in the shop," she recalls. "My mom and dad were fussy about everything being just so. No crumbs, no dirt, you know." Mrs. Blackburn adjusts the pearl comb that holds her thick French twist in place.

"Kathleen?" the director nods her head.

"One sister. She died. Of pneumonia. Two years old. Tore us all apart. You can imagine the state my mother was in."

"What else, Kathleen?"

"I was spoiled rotten after that. I enjoyed it. Actually, I still do!" Kathleen's memory has been jarred. "I had five babies!"

"Was it scary having your first baby, Kathleen?" the director asks.

"Oh no! I was too excited," she shouts. "She was gorgeous. She had black hair and purple eyes. Died of pneumonia at the age of two."

"Faye, what can you tell us about your family?"

"Oh," she begins, embarrassed. "I'd have to get a diagram. I can't remember who was in my family right off."

"Hmm!" Kathleen says. "Can't remember her relatives! What on earth. How can you forget such a thing?" She turns to whisper into the ear of the boy still sitting silently beside her. "Sometimes old people are funnier than young people. In fact, most of the time!"

Kathleen, spoiled but charming still, has more to say. "I used to have a golden dog named Farney. That's my nickname. We had a harbor. A boat. We'd haul it out. It was great."

Faye remembers something and interrupts. "I *did* have a brother! I remember now. I wrote him a letter during the war. 'I wish you'd come home so I could look at you.'"

Angie cannot quiz the others in the room. They have nothing to say because they have forgotten everything. It is all gone now. It never happened.

·4·

I always thought my father looked like Richard M. Nixon.

It doesn't surprise me to find my mother one day rubbing her hands over a picture of the former president in a Sunday magazine. It's a photo that accompanies one of the many long pieces commemorating his recent death.

My mother notices Sam sitting off to one side, alone, hooked up to an oxygen tank. His complexion is as gray as his hair. His face is unshaved and his mouth is open in sleep. She rises to join him. She caresses his head. She adjusts his hose (I follow close along to repair her damage). And then, suddenly, she turns away and drags me with her.

We sit. She places her hand on the picture of Nixon, then my hand on top of hers, and hers on top of mine. I complete the pattern. She sends a playful, toothless grin in my direction. We rest together like tired children in the middle of the afternoon, and I notice her eyes redden as they begin to close.

In the background, a basketball game is on the television. A play by Shaquille O'Neal of the Magic brings fans to their feet.

·5·

The last time my mother saw my father was at Akron City Hospital. My father was dying, dying of a lung tumor made from the harsh ingredients of his seventy-nine years: the tar and nicotine of thousands of cigarettes, the Pennsylvania coal dust he inhaled as a boy, the lampblack he breathed in every day of his forty-year career in the plants of the Rubber Capital of the World. He could barely breathe without oxygen. One of his lungs had been sucked into a bottle to prevent it from filling again with fluid, and powdered with a substance that glued it shut forever. His chest rose and fell in sobs.

My mother could not stay still in her chair. She had few words left and was delusional now the better part of most days. But she sensed something very awful was about to happen. She tugged at Tom Coyne's sheets, covered his legs (which he would immediately uncover, it was summer and warm even in air conditioning), stroked his thick hair which had lost its beautiful curl and all of its luster since his illness. She would straighten his table (beyond recognition), accidentally pull his oxygen loose, tie and retie his gown in knots no nurse could unsnarl.

And then, exhausted by her labors, she sat down beside me. With words not really meant for anyone—not for me, not for her husband, not even for herself—she constructed the last truly complete sentence I would ever hear her utter. "Tommy," she said in a voice abnormally loud, intensified by her deafness, "you aren't going to make it!" She was right. My father laughed.

Somehow my father knew then that it was all right to die. She had let him go. She had given permission.

·6·

My son visits with me when he comes home from school. He sits with his grandmother and holds her hand and tries to talk about something he imagines she might remember. Annabelle does not know him. But sometimes I think I see her tip her head slightly when my son's loud and rich voice, so much like Thomas Coyne's, touches her deaf ears.

Once in early winter, near Christmas, we walked my mother back and forth, up and down the halls, over and over in the same monotonous pattern we had so many times before. Except for our absolute silence, we could have been carolers, bundled up in coats and sweaters and boots and heavy socks.

She suddenly stopped in front of a room not her own. She took my hand, dropping my son's, and led me inside. She left me there and made it clear by her outstretched arm that I was not to follow this time. She returned to my son, faced him, drew her arms around his neck, and rested her head on his chest. She stroked his thick curly hair.

My son's long arms dangled in surprise. Slowly, he pressed them to her back, as a lover would, and rocked her in his arms.

·7·

"William D. Nevel. That's 'N-e-v-e-l.' I've been waiting over a year for him," the woman in green complains. "I want him home next to me. Where he belongs."

Benny walks over to her and tells her to shut up. He seems disgusted by her shrill voice and strong will.

"Come here," she orders Benny, pointing a stern finger. He obeys. She rises majestically from her chair and gestures for him to sit.

"You sit there for my Bill. Take a load off your figure. Sit. It's your Bill too, you know. We can both see the door."

Benny sits. She pulls a chair beside him and sits again. Her posture is perfect and straight. One arm holds tightly to the top of her cane, forming a ninety degree angle with her body. " 'N-e-v-e-l,' " she spells once more. "That's my husband's name. And it's my name too. He'll come. I know he'll come. Let's wait."

In early spring, a miracle occurred.

In front of The Woods is an artificial pond. Every spring geese arrive and take up residence. Gulls visit from the lake across the road. Glossy-headed drakes and mottled brown hens begin to patrol the perimeter of the pond. The birds are beautiful and always a surprise. But they were not the miracle this year.

In early April, as I turned the corner of the drive from the street, I saw two long, slender shafts of neck lift high above the water. They were white, not mottled tan. They were piercingly white. A snow goose, I thought.

After I parked my car, I hurried to the edge of the recessed pond. Two gracefully curved necks ending in orange-red bills with odd black knobs looped in my direction. They were swans. Mute swans. There were two of them, one slightly smaller than the other. Their tails tilted upward, regally.

There they were, two elegant swans, sailing across a small pond in front of a building where people went to hide, or to be hidden, or to die. There they were in the most unlikely spot imaginable on earth, in all their troubling presence.

That night, they floated up in my dreams and spoke to me. Their bills opened slowly and their eyes stared into mine. But I could not understand what they had to say. They spoke a language I did not speak, in sounds as soft as the feathers on their necks, as soft as my mother's palms. I listened harder, and then harder still, afraid that they would never speak to me again. But I could not, no matter how I tried, translate a single word. And then they stopped, grew silent, and flew away.

CHAPTER TWO

❧

Words

"When he signs a check, I can tell he's not really
writing. He's drawing a picture of his name, that's all,
and that picture's going to be the next thing to go—"
A. G. MOJTABAI, *Called Out*

·1·

Mabel. I walk through the nursing wing and see her sitting in a new room, looking smaller than ever in her wheelchair. Queen for a Day, she sits on a metal throne, tufts of hair blazing white, a polka-dotted ribbon keeping white curls from falling into her face. She has been moved from Tanglewood and taken to the nursing wing. Probably a fall. A fall so often precedes the mysterious disappearance of a resident from Tanglewood. If nursing is needed, Tanglewood residents are moved. That's how it works.

I miss Mabel when I arrive at Tanglewood. I miss her mischievous smile. "Yoo-hooo!" she would frequently screech, waving her hand in the air, wanting attention from anyone who would give it.

"What do you want, Mabel?" the first person free would yell across the room.

"Something. Cheerful. Help!"

Mabel always would be reading an old issue of *Good Housekeeping*. She would turn the pages and stare at pictures of beautiful interiors, perfect gardens, luscious food.

Sometimes I saw her lick her lips.

·2·

Only a few words remain. She will chatter occasionally, but not much. "Yeah . . . cause . . . may." She looks puzzled. I answer. "It will be all right, Mother." I kiss her cheek. She rolls her eyes and nods. A short time later, she tilts her head and puzzles over something else.

We walk to the door of the patio on a warm, rainy afternoon. "Water," she says looking outside. "Water," she says, pointing to the dripping leaves. There is no doubt. She really has found the word. She is coming back to me. Just a word, but she is in my world. I'm sure of it.

She pulls my arm and we walk toward her room. She looks at my shoes and suddenly drops to her hands and knees. Creeping slowly around my loafers, she digs her index finger into the sides, the heels. She kisses the tongue and rests her cheek on the soft brown leather. She presses her hands to the carpet and her veins knot in huge lumps, like blue West Virginia coal.

She smiles up at me, gums bright with moisture. She rises, dizzy.

·3·

Butterflies made of colored paper recently appeared on the doors of every resident. They were obviously made in a Vacation Bible School class somewhere in town. The wings of my mother's butterfly are bright yellow, decorated with pink smudges.

The body of the butterfly is black. A white oval has been glued to the middle of each body—probably by the teacher. And on the oval is a typed message from the Book of Psalms.

My mother's message is this: "Be strong and take heart, all you who hope in the Lord."

Could the child who colored around the words, the teacher who typed them, or even the psalmist who wrote them in the first place have had any idea what they really meant? The woman behind the door lives in a world without words, in a world where language has largely disappeared, a world full of only silence, of wild gibberish, of screams that cut my heart in two.

The psalmist cannot, dare not, advise her any longer with words. He cannot touch her. He, too, even he, would fall silent in her presence. She would heal him of his arrogance. Still him forever. Heal him and still him forever and forever.

·4·

In 1989 my son and I joined my father and mother at Bob Evans Farms Restaurant for breakfast. We did this often. My father needed as much of us as he could get. I understood this only later, after he died.

In the restaurant that day, my mother spotted an ordinary housefly inside the window next to her. She was delighted. Letters and syllables scrambled electrically in front of her, in front of us all. What *was* that creature? She looked for clues on placemats, salt and pepper shakers, utensils. She looked everywhere except toward our lips. She was proud and wanted to name the thing alone.

Suddenly, she yelled with pleasure. "A pepper bird!"

We smiled at the occasional wonder of the disease. At the perpetual wonder of my mother.

·5·

"What's new, Millie?" I ask.

She looks confused and moves her tongue rapidly over her

lips. She surprises herself as she stares down at the page-length ad in the newspaper on her lap.

"Forty-Eight-Hour Sale!" she screams as her finger flutters across the page like the pointer of a Geiger counter.

·6·

My mother read more but wrote less than my father. She never sent many letters. If she did, they were brief. When she mailed a special occasion card to anyone, usually only her signature was attached—no note. Even sympathy cards would be signed without the expected flourish of emotion: "With sympathy, Annabelle Coyne." That was all. She always *said* what she had to say, often quickly, always directly. A few words sufficed.

In the spring of 1986, the spring of their fiftieth wedding anniversary, my father and mother took a cross-country car trip. Neither of them had ever been West. It was a second honeymoon, the trip of a lifetime.

They started out on I-71 to Louisville, Kentucky, took I-65 to Nashville, and then picked up I-40 across Tennessee, Arkansas, Oklahoma, Texas, New Mexico, and Arizona—all the way to the Pacific Ocean. From Los Angeles they traveled up the coast on U.S. 101. Near the Oregon/Washington border, they veered over to Portland, then took I-5 to British Columbia. They spun through Canada on Canada Route 1 across the rest of British Columbia, Alberta, Saskatchewan, Manitoba, Ontario, Quebec, clear over to Montreal. There they crossed the border back to the United States and rolled south onto I-87 to Albany. They returned on I-90 to Ohio six weeks after they had set out. My mother and father had traveled over seven thousand miles together.

Across coffee and toast the morning after their return, Annabelle stared with annoyance into my father's eyes, eyes red from days and days of fighting the road. "Tommy," she said, "you never take me anywhere."

·7·

In 1986 my mother wrote the only letter I ever received from her in my life, probably prodded to do so by my father. It was a thank you for their fiftieth wedding anniversary party that my family and I had held for my parents in July.

Dear Joyce, Dan, and Steve:
Sending a letter to both of you and Steve. All of you worked so hard, I don't know how you managed it. Thanks so much for everything. As Tommy said, "What a day—what a party." A big "Thank You" from all of us.

Annabell and Tom
X X X

Ironically, her only letter to me confirmed the onset of her terrible illness, an onset we all were trying hard not to notice. Words were crossed out, "all of us" oddly crept in where "both of us" belonged. And my mother left off the "e" in Annabelle. She was forgetting how to spell her own name. She was packing her bags and heading for a country called Aphasia.

Besides this letter, I have only one other piece of writing from my mother. I don't even remember what occasion it commemorates. But on a white florist's card, now yellow at the edges, are these spare words, scripted by Edna Annabelle Haberkost Coyne: "Congratulations, Darling. Mother & Dad."

I roll the words in my mouth like diamonds.

CHAPTER THREE

∾

Plaques and Tangles

This is madness, I think. "This is madness," I say out loud. But I know better. This is Alzheimer's disease.
MARION ROACH, *Another Name for Madness*

·1·

Tanglewood is a tiny and simple world, but still a world far too complicated for most of the people living here. A thousand times a day, residents of Tanglewood ask where their rooms are and where they sit for dinner. Names printed in black marker and pasted to bright backgrounds appear on dining room tables, on doors of rooms, above beds. The construction-paper backgrounds are color-coded. Each resident has become a Crayola crayon in a box of twenty-four. My mother's color is consistently, always, purple.

A long table runs across one side of the living area. A heavy piece of glass protects its surface, but also weighs down a photograph display of residents. Their names are printed boldly on strips of paper taped above each picture. A banner appears at the top: "Seniors at Tanglewood. Summer 1994."

Mr. Miller just arrived at Tanglewood and still knows his name, and where he eats, and how to find his room. Mr. Miller always wears his baseball cap tightly on his head to keep his brains from spilling out and says the same thing a hundred times a day to anyone who will listen. "Have you seen Sandra Miller? Tell her I'm looking for her."

But for residents who no longer can read, or have forgotten their names, the signs become useless. Lost men and women sit at tables and with thick yellow thumbnails pick and scratch the heavy tape that bolts their names to the furniture.

· 2 ·

When I arrived for an early winter visit in 1994, I noticed that my mother seemed to have something tucked in her pants. Her slender waist and small stomach protruded in unnatural ridges. I pulled the elastic waistband toward me and heard the sound of fabric slapping plastic. My mother was wearing a diaper, a Depend brief for adults.

She was becoming occasionally incontinent. This had not been a good week for her; there had been many accidents. For some time now, an aide had been taking her to the bathroom every four hours. But even that wasn't working. Annabelle had forgotten what a toilet was, after using one for over eighty years.

She would sit on the cold seat, but would no longer understand the purpose for being there. She could not urinate on command. Her body processes were beyond her control. Sometimes she would refuse to cooperate altogether, scream "No!" and strike the arms and chests of attendants who were trying to pull her pants down or help her bend her knees and crouch.

When I visit my mother, I am keenly aware of urination. I check immediately to see if she is in a Depend or wearing her own underpants. We visit her toilet several times, and once in a while she understands what to do. If I use the toilet first in front of her, she seems to show more interest.

Once she guided me into a room not her own, and stood for ten minutes staring directly at the toilet bowl. Like a bird discovering a new birdbath in a somewhat familiar garden, she angled her head several times in confusion. Then, she clasped the safety rail on one side with her left hand and leaned over slightly to flick the water in the bowl with her right. Finally, she turned around, backed in, pulled down her pants, sat, and peed.

I saw her grin as she closed her eyes.

· 3 ·

There are many varieties of dementia. Alzheimer's is just one. My mother also suffers from multi-infarct, known as mixed dementia. At least three times since being admitted to Tanglewood, she has had "transient ischemic attacks," or TIAs, temporary warning signs of possible stroke. On two such occasions, she just passed out at dinner, fell off her chair and onto the floor. I always race to the unit after receiving calls about these episodes, but when I arrive my mother is usually sitting quietly in her seat, unaware that anything unusual has happened.

Often she is smiling, perhaps secretly proud that nothing so minor will ever take her from this earth. Alzheimer's is the opponent she must fear, the opponent worthy of my mother—not some feeble villain of the vascular system.

I know a stroke will never kill her. I know it for a fact.

· 4 ·

Famous people who have died from Alzheimer's disease: Norman Rockwell, Sugar Ray Robinson, Edmund O'Brien, Rita Hayworth, Otto Preminger, E. B. White, Ross McDonald, Joyce

Chen. Famous people who have cared for someone with Alzheimer's: Mike Myers, Jay Rockefeller, Angie Dickinson, Keith Hernandez, Deborah Hoffmann, Shelley Fabares, Nancy Reagan. Lewis Thomas called it a "disease-of-the-century." He said, "It is the worst of all diseases, not just for what it does to the patient, but for its devastating effects on families and friends." Thomas singled it out in 1980 as the one disease that ought to be targeted by the government for special research funding. He urged private foundations that currently have a large stake in the "Health-Care Delivery System" to commit half their endowments to research on senile dementia, knowing the government cannot handle this disease alone.

No one can.

·5·

My mother was diagnosed with Alzheimer's when she was seventy-six years old. She visited the doctor, much against her will, and was given an MSQ (mental-status questionnaire examination) and a CAT scan. "DAT," her diagnosis read. Dementia of the Alzheimer Type. Profound brain atrophy.

Due to the late onset of her disease, I am not at extremely great risk.

But I am at higher risk than others, and I know it.

No physical symptom that mimics brain atrophy is casual to me. If I feel my head cloud from a headache or heat, I picture brain cells dying behind my eyes. When I misplace a folder or show the slightest hesitancy about finding my parked car—or a word, especially a word—I panic.

Sometimes I think I will kill myself if I find out this is my fate.

But maybe I will not.

I used to ask my father how he did all he did, how he, a very impatient man by nature, stood the tension and demands of my mother's illness with such humor and grace. "She's like an old dog," he would say. "I've gotten kind of used to her over the years."

My mother's illness has been both the greatest task she has ever asked of me, and the greatest gift she has ever given. It has broken me in half, and made me whole in a way I could never have been without it. It has destroyed me completely, but healed me for all eternity. How can I explain such remarkable contradictions?

Her illness made my father a great man. A truly great man whom I came to adore.

As brutal and incomprehensible as it might sound, even to me, perhaps most especially to me, I think I would let it happen, should it happen to me.

·6·

Since my mother entered Stage 3 of her disease, the final stage, the following drugs have been prescribed: Ativan, Thorazine, milk of magnesia, Darvocet, aspirin, estrogen, Senokot syrup, Sinequan, Provera, and Thera-M vitamins. She has been on doses of Thorazine as high as 75 mg, when severely agitated, and as low as 10 mg. She took her first dose of Thorazine in 1993, for "obsessiveness, compulsiveness, hitting, kicking, psychotic behaviors." I am always told when the dosage is upped or lowered. And I am never happier than when my mother is on only 10 mg. Or on none at all.

Other drugs that those with Alzheimer's have been given include Hydergine, Cognex, Haldol, Stelazine, Compazine, choline combined with lecithin, and neuropeptides. Eldepryl, originally prescribed for Parkinson's disease, seems to increase sociability in people with Alzheimer's, but results are inconclusive. Ibuprofen, the drug contained in such pain relievers as Advil, Motrin, and Nuprin, has been the promising focus of a fourteen-year Johns Hopkins University study. It seems to reduce the risk of developing Alzheimer's disease by as much as 30 to 60 percent. And tacrine, now approved for sale, as well as Exelon, a promising drug currently being tested, shows evidence of slowing or temporarily reversing the disease.

Lamps continue to flicker late into the night at research centers throughout the world, looking for magic.

·7·

The county where my mother resides reports 8,517 cases of Alzheimer's disease. In the region where she lives, 50,000 people are afflicted with Alzheimer's, enough to fill a football stadium. In the state that Annabelle Coyne has always called home, in the state where my mother will live out her life and be buried beside my father when she dies, 170,944 people are gradually losing their minds.

·8·

If you were to board a hovercraft and fly over two human brains, one normal and one diseased by Alzheimer's, you would notice some remarkable differences.

If you had a giant PET scanner with you, an imager built for the gods, the AD brain would exhibit huge oceans of purple in the center, not healthy green or turquoise islands. Purple shows fluid in the brain, fluid that increases as more and more brain cells die. When you return, you'll never like purple again. You will fold your priestly robes into a cedar chest and leave the order. You will avoid grape jelly the rest of your life.

The normal brain has folds in the cerebrum called *sulci*. They are narrow and shallow. But a brain diseased by Alzheimer's exhibits deeper valleys, and much wider. The valleys widen as the brain shrinks. Neurons lose their intricate branches and fill up with abnormal protein deposits, called tangles. Outside the nerve cells plaques form, graveyards for dead or dying neurons.

The disease has built a labyrinth from which no one can ever escape. It has gouged out the brain with a forklift. Even without your scanner you can see the valleys of death.

You could drop a huge silver ball into one of the wide crevices of an Alzheimer's brain from your craft and never find it again. It would roll forever in the pinball machine from hell.

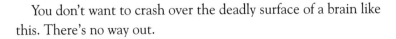

You don't want to crash over the deadly surface of a brain like this. There's no way out.

·9·

Frances moves in perpetual motion. She sits in her wheel-chair and shakes from the top of her right shoulder to the little toe of her right foot. She is in an uncontrollable flutter. She is a seventeen-year locust, incapable of producing sound except through the constant movement of her wings.

The parts of her brain that control her muscles are being destroyed, day by day, cell by cell. She has tangles from Alzheimer's, and tangles from progressive palsy. Frances's brain is all knotted up.

And so is Reggie's.

Reggie is constantly on parade, wearing a T-shirt that says "Over the Hill" and marching rigidly over the same ground every day. He seems practically paralyzed—and is. He can move his lower body, but his arms are as inflexible and rigid as a man-nequin's. His hands clump in fists and his fingers seem to have disappeared into his palms. His features are as fixed as those on the face of a coin. Nothing ever moves—not eyebrows, lips, not even skin. In the four years I have known him, his expression has never changed.

Reggie belongs on Mount Rushmore with Washington, Jefferson, Lincoln, and Theodore Roosevelt.

I sometimes wonder what Reggie was doing when his face decided to turn to stone.

·10·

A phone message is on my answering machine when I arrive home from a morning of errands. It's Esther's. "Now, don't worry," she begins. And then, the terrifying words I dread even spoken in Esther's calm tones, "But your mother . . ."

My mother had been standing behind a rocker, watching a small group dance to music during an activity period. She had lost consciousness and fallen to her knees, her hands still clinging firmly to the back of the chair. Nurses rushed to her side. She quickly snapped awake and allowed herself to be guided to a sofa. They observed her for half an hour. Then, as she lifted herself up, the nurses holding tightly to her arms, her entire right side, and her left arm, began to twitch. Her body jerked uncontrollably in a fit of seizure—an occasional twist to the disease that appears in late stages. She began a horrible dance, a Saint Vitus dance, a dance that can only be danced alone.

Esther sat my mother in a G/C, a geriatric chair that restricts movement, and began to administer oxygen. She pulled the chair beside her at the nurse's station. She had called my mother's doctor and been advised to monitor her carefully for one hour and summon an ambulance if my mother did not improve or respond.

For one hour, Annabelle stared into space, unable to follow a face or a finger trying to pull her back to Tanglewood. She twisted and jerked to music no one else heard. Completely gone, she permitted the oxygen mask to remain in place, for exactly one hour. Then, almost as if a timer had been set in her dead head, my mother tore the mask from her face, blinked her eyes, smiled slyly at the aides and nurses gathered lovingly around her, and skipped away down the hall.

Once more, she had evaded her executioner.

·11·

Victoria likes to sit by the TV. Not because she likes TV but because she likes to pull hard on the steel cart that supports it. Victoria's hands are like yard clippers, like Venus flytraps. They grab and pinch and pull and tear whatever they can reach.

She sits in a vinyl chair, rolling up her turquoise pants far above her knees. Victoria has beautiful legs, and perhaps she remembers this about herself. Her calves are muscular and have not discolored and bulged out with veins like those of the rest of the women in the unit.

She is busy today. She takes a Kleenex and stuffs it in the toe of her slipper, pushing the slipper almost out of reach—but not quite. Fetch the Slipper is her favorite game. She supports herself on the arms of the chair and tries to rise. But her beautiful legs no longer know what to do. Dim signals sent out by her brain are returned marked "Address Unknown." She raises her rear six inches off the vinyl and then drops back to her sitting position. Again and again, a hundred times an hour, she tries to rise but invariably falls back into her seat.

Her only other movement is to grab hold of blouses, shirts, TV carts, arms, anything that she might trap. She has torn sleeves off uniforms, ripped fabric belts from waists, scratched forearms, and upset juice carts. Victoria is strong and quick. If she has you in her vise, you must strain to free yourself. And when you do, and run away, she howls and sobs like a little child.

The nurses gently scold her, but know there will be no remembering. There is no point to a reprimand. When they lift her from her seat into a wheelchair, they swiftly grab her under the arms and let her flail like a spider. She points her arms high into the air, turning thumbs and index fingers into pistols, laughs wildly, and tongues a sound.

"Da-da-da-da-daaa!" she repeats over and over, shooting the demons that have done this to her.

·12·

In the late spring of 1994, I discovered that my mother had forgotten not only her bladder but also her bowels. We were sitting outside in the patio on a cool day when I realized how foreign her own body had become to her.

She suddenly grew extremely restless. She began pacing the walk. Then she went to each corner of the enclosure and pressed her right shoulder firmly against it. She proceeded to rub her body up and down the seams of the building, up and down the bricks and boards.

Finally she stopped her frenzied activity at the fourth corner, the corner where Tanglewood abuts the nursing wing. She pushed her back hard against the bricks and bent her legs slightly. Her face flushed. She looked at me in terror. I tried to pull her toward the Tanglewood entrance, but she stood stiff and immovable.

Slowly, she took her right hand and slid it inside the back of her sweatpants. She brought it out after a few moments, heaped with her own warm excrement. I had no idea what to do.

Shaking, I grabbed a tissue from my purse, but she would not release her grasp and let me remove the waste. Instead, she began throwing it against windows and walls and white doors. It was everywhere and she wouldn't stop until it was all gone. Her hand was colored brown and under her nails were pieces of feces. But at last she let me clasp her wrist and clean her.

It was then that I asked the nurses about her bowel habits. They said this had been going on for several weeks. They were not surprised and told me it was common in the late stages of the disease. I was not to be alarmed. It was normal.

In the unit itself, they would find pieces of my mother's excrement in the grooves of wooden handrails (her favorite hiding place), in corners, on light bulbs. Once they smelled it at night warmed by the glow of a lamp. Another time they found steaming coils on a wool welcome mat I had bought my mother for Christmas. It was woven with the words "Home Sweet Home."

On one occasion she had proudly placed a neatly formed ball of it on the counter of the nurse's station and stuck a pencil she had found unguarded smack in the center, like a birthday cake for a one-year-old.

CHAPTER FOUR

Nurses and Staff

*If there is wisdom to be found, it must be in the
knowledge that human beings are capable of the kind
of love and loyalty that transcends not only the
physical debasement but even the spiritual weariness
of the years of sorrow.*

SHERWIN B. NULAND,
"Alzheimer's Disease," from *How We Die*

·1·

Carolyn is huffing down the hall toward Tanglewood. I see her flowered blouse, her trademark, a mile away. She has a piece of paper in her hand loaded with signatures.

"Have you been reading about Walt Disney?" she asks me as we approach the unit together, her glasses slipping down her nose. "Disney is trying to build near Manassas. I have a petition already completed. They can't do that. This is sacred, hallowed ground!"

I agree, and hold the door for her as she enters Tanglewood in front of me.

·2·

Mrs. Goldman. Admitted in February of 1994. Mrs. Goldman is a small woman, the matriarch of the unit at ninety-nine years. "Ninety-nine," she says to anyone who will listen. "It's better to go earlier. Good Lord."

Mrs. Goldman sits on a chair upholstered in dark pink vinyl. A chair that gives her a view of nearly everything that's going on. She can see the television screen in the central area by leaning just inches to her left. Even without leaning she can hear the sound of Vivien Leigh pleading with Clark Gable on a video of *Gone With the Wind*, one of the unit's favorite films. "Oh, Rhett. I'm so cold and hungry."

She sits with her walker in front of her, dressed as she dressed thirty years, fifty years, seventy years ago. "My husband did this to me. He always was good to me. I don't understand. He thinks I can't take care of myself and do the shopping. You never know when you get old what will happen. I had a beautiful house."

An aide stops to listen. She strokes Mrs. Goldman's hair. "You're entitled to your opinion, Mrs. Goldman. Everyone is."

·3·

"Relax," says Esther. "Just relax, Stanley."

Stanley is in a wheelchair, shaking all over. He wears a fleece sweat suit, the typical attire of both men and women in Tanglewood. They look like dabs of primary color, Olympic athletes, gumdrops: purple, black, turquoise, red mounds of cotton and Spandex. Stanley is dressed in Reebok tennis shoes and bright gold sweats—the Golden Fleece of Tanglewood. A nervous aide is trying to push him as quickly as she can toward his room and his private bath. But Stanley drags his feet and nearly topples head first onto the floor.

He winces, moans, then screams. "Can't hold it!"

Esther quietly, powerfully, rises from her seat behind the nurse's station and places her hand on the arm of Stanley's chair.

"Relax," she exhales. She rests her hand on his stomach, close to the groin. She lifts his feet that have been scuffing across the close-napped carpet and slides them onto the footrests she locks in place. "Relax, Stan," she smiles.

He stops shaking. The aide continues her brief journey down the hall to Stanley's room.

·4·

Esther is from West Virginia. She loves the mountains. She loves her religion. She loves the hymns sung by visiting church groups.

Esther works the day shift and has been at The Woods twenty-five years, five of those at Tanglewood. She is one of the founders who argued for a special wing for people like my mother. When Esther is on duty, the residents are spoiled. They know it and they love it.

Esther doesn't mind spills or messes. In the four years I've been coming to Tanglewood, I've never seen her irritated, annoyed, short-tempered. Once I saw an angry resident punch Esther in the stomach because Esther was trying to lift her from her chair so that her diaper could be changed. Esther caught her breath and then looked directly in her enemy's eye. "Dana," Esther said, in the tone of a strict but loving parent, "no more. That's enough. Come with me. It's over." The woman nodded her head and echoed Esther's last words, "Come with me. It's over." She walked with Esther, hand in hand, down the hall.

Esther always has a story to tell me about Annabelle when I arrive. She loves my mother. I hope my mother dies during her shift.

·5·

I stand near the nurse's station talking with Esther. I place my elbow on the counter and rest my chin in the palm of my right hand and listen to her voice. It nearly rocks me to sleep. She tells me about her vacation. She'll be going to a special Florida beach with her grandson, she says, where the sand is always cool, like baking powder from a red tin can, not like sand at all.

As she talks, three male residents drift to the counter like ghosts. They stand side by side, arms folded, staring at Esther—much as I am.

"They think this is a bar," she laughs. She pats, then squeezes, each of the six hands. The men turn, almost in step, and say something about cars and sons and keys in a half-human roar. They lower their heads like Minotaurs and waddle down a leg of their labyrinth looking for something they will never find because they have forgotten what it is.

·6·

My mother quickly grabs an unattended piece of paper from the counter top of the nurse's station. She folds it three times and then leads me toward the patio. It will be my task the rest of the afternoon to recover the sheet and return it to the nurse on duty when I leave.

We sit under the umbrella table and relax. My mother smiles and stares at me with blue clouded eyes, eyes so much like the sky today that it is remarkable. She looks at her right hand and is surprised to see the paper that she holds. She unfolds it and tries to read, but can only growl, "Gee, yee, gee." She shrugs her shoulders, refolds the paper, and places it tightly in my hand. She laughs and stares off somewhere else.

I open the paper and start to iron it back to its original condition with my hand. I look down at it as my fingers try to heal the spectacular folds my mother has created, and read:

All Nurses and Nurses' Aides
Please Plan to Come.

Inservice
June 28, 1994
HOSPICE
Comfort-Oriented Care for the Dying
7:00 A.M.
2:00 P.M.
3:00 P.M.

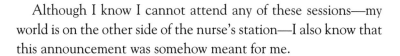

Although I know I cannot attend any of these sessions—my world is on the other side of the nurse's station—I also know that this announcement was somehow meant for me.

·7·

Carolyn comes in at 3:00 P.M. She seldom arrives without something for the unit. A small box of her discarded books, flowered blouses frayed at the sleeves or collar, records from the '50s, a huge blossom of one sort or another from her garden of perennials.

When Carolyn takes a break, you'll find her reading in the lounge, enjoying a cup of coffee. She reads the works of the good writers.

Carolyn loves the difficult evening hours right after supper best. She will gather people around her by the record player and the bookshelves. Sometimes she'll read to them from children's books. Or she'll tell them a story that she told her own children years before.

She knows exactly what popular songs residents loved when they were young, and she plays them on the turntable. "Remember that, Fannie?" she'll ask with excitement. Occasionally a word from a familiar refrain, always from the refrain, is recovered by a resident. One person listens to a collection of Gershwin songs and yells, " 'S won-der-ful!" The person next to her surprises herself by chiming in " 'S mar-ve-lous!" Carolyn cries "Good!" and sings the whole line: " 'S won-der-ful!——'S mar-vel-ous!——You should care——for me!"

But the good cheer soon fades. The residents lose interest. They grow restless and begin to rub foreheads and become angry for no reason other than a missed beat in their brains, for no reason other than the sun is going down. Carolyn reads the cues quickly, glides to the nurse's closet, locates a small black case, and returns to her stage.

Some residents recognize the case and become still. They smile and hold each other's hands. A few who remember applaud. They look at the long case and the two shiny locks on its edge.

33

Carolyn snaps the locks open and removes the pieces of a silver flute. She assembles it, wets her lips, and trills.

·8·

Al works the evening shift. He arrives at Tanglewood around 3:00 P.M. and stays to 11:00 P.M. Al loves sports, especially baseball. He walks with a mild limp, and smiles easily. He takes care of the men in the unit, lifting them, carrying them to restrooms and beds and dinner tables. He sets the tables himself sometimes, helps change the linen on the beds and the towels in the bathrooms. He tightens Benny's bowling suspenders and zips up pants. He is a strong man.

"Are you OK, Mr. Miller?" you'll hear him say. And you'll see him sit among the men and talk or laugh, or be silent with them, as they choose.

He asks Stanley who will win the game on Saturday. He flips a rubber baseball in his right hand. His language is as simple as the language the residents speak.

Sometimes, before dinner, music is played to a circle of listeners, the way it was when my mother's seizure occurred. Al becomes a prince. He makes women forget they cannot walk. They throw their canes into a heap. He magically lifts ancient bodies formerly soldered to wheelchairs into his arms and ballroom dances to the music on the record player.

Color comes into the cheeks of the women for just a minute. Someone hits a balloon into the air. A toast is made with pineapple juice in pill cups.

The music winds to an end and the needle scratches its finale. The women move more slowly once again and begin their search through a pile of walkers and canes for something to hold them up.

·9·

On July 30, 1988, my parents visited me in Boone, North Carolina. I was there for a month-long seminar. We had difficulty locating a restaurant close by, so we traveled to Blowing Rock up the road and entered the Green Park Inn. It seemed like a mistake at first. The prices were high and the whole idea of the place different from what my family was used to. Clearly this was a spot for rich people from the Piedmont. The women were manicured and jeweled; the men, right out of Fitzgerald novels, were dressed in cool linen suits. They came to hold one another and to dance to the live big band music paid for by the restaurant's high prices.

But soon all of that moved to the background. Things shifted when I heard my father ask Annabelle to dance.

It was now the summer of their fifty-second wedding anniversary. She was not even sure where she was when my father extended his hand to her in the Green Park Inn. Before we had gone to dinner, she had proudly shown me around her motel room and talked about her "new house." We had examined gleaming tile, closets, Kleenex dispensers, velvet paintings in red and black, and bed quilts with wide bars of color. When she left the motel, she grew frightened, and absolutely still.

"Will you dance with me, Annabelle?" he asked, lifting her from her chair, his great buck teeth lighting the way through the dark, like headlights.

She looked alarmed, but trusted him, knowing she had no strength but his. They walked arm in arm to the dance floor. He stood erect, remembering other days. My mother softly placed her hand in his and rested her arm across the collar of his cheap white shirt.

He pumped his arms up and down as the music began, and exaggerated his steps like a mechanical monkey to help my mother follow. But it was too difficult for her. Once a graceful dancer, my mother no longer could keep her feet from becoming tangled and she started to pull away. Her body did not remember enough anymore. It remembered something, but not enough for the Green Park Inn.

Without pausing, my father leaned over and bent softly to the ground. He lifted my mother's right foot and placed it on top his left. Then as he stood, he raised her body gently until her left foot rested on his other shoe. They danced for over an hour like that. He carried her on his feet, carried her full weight, carried her like a swan carries a cygnet on its back.

They danced to "Alice Blue Gown." I could hear my father humming loudly off key whenever the sound of the band dimmed. I unconsciously began to mouth the words of the refrain, words as common in our house as "The Lord's Prayer" and "The Star-Spangled Banner." Words you saluted, or stood at attention for. "Till it wilt-ed I wore it, I'll al-ways a-dore it, My sweet lit-tle A-lice blue gown."

They danced as they had danced at Summit Beach Park and the East Market Center when they were young. They danced with eyes closed, my father helping his wife remember the fun of being young, the inevitable connection between a saxophone and your feet, the feel of warm bodies close together. Once I saw him whisper in one of her deaf ears. Across the room, I may have heard her laugh.

·10·

Esther brings some apple juice to the woman in green. She strokes Gloria's henna hair and buttons the cuffs of her blouse. Esther yawns leisurely and turns. "You're lovely," Gloria shouts in Esther's direction. "Keep it that *way*. I don't mean north and south. I mean the way you are."

·11·

Maggy works in the nursing wing but sometimes substitutes in Tanglewood. "I watch your mother in the patio out the window of my wing," she tells me as she coaxes Annabelle to take her medicines, buried in applesauce and frozen yogurt. "She picks in the soil, rips up weeds and things. Did she have a garden?"

"A small garden," I say. "She was wonderful, really."

"Still is," Maggy corrects me.

A young aide chimes in. "Annabelle was mad at me yesterday, weren't you, Annabelle?" The aide throws her lower lip into a pout and my mother laughs and pats the girl's face with her hand. "She took her supper outside and I made her come in. She was getting red as a beet and I worried she'd faint. She's my favorite person in the unit because she's so feisty." I suddenly remember the first day we admitted my mother. She pretended to know all the people who warmly greeted her. But after she realized that something was wrong, she ran to the patio and tried to throw herself over the fence, bloodying her arms and legs.

The aide seems to be dreaming, just as I am. "She's so spunky," she continues, talking more to herself than anyone else. "I can see myself being like her when I'm old. I'd *like* to be like her." I feel as if this young aide and I have secretly formed a pact, pricked our fingers together and become blood sisters for the remainder of our lives.

"She had me late in life," I tell Maggy, just making conversation after the young aide drifts dreamlike toward another resident. "Doctors told her that with one ovary there would be little chance of children. It was a myth, of course, but she believed it and it almost came true. At nearly forty, there I was."

"Then you're a miracle!"

"Yes," I reply. "I guess I'm a miracle."

·12·

Jackie pulls a chair beside us. "She's doing fine," she whispers. "I know it's not easy. But you calm her."

I feel the hot tears swell in my eyes and look away. I can't even thank her for saying this. Jackie sits with us, in the hurry of the middle of her afternoon. She sits and sits, as if she's invited us both to her home for lemonade in the summer when there's nothing else to do.

"Your mother has so much energy. What did she do when she was young?" Jackie asks.

And I tell her the story of my mother, who was different from other women, different without even knowing it, without my even knowing it then.

"I can see that in her even now," she says when I finish. "I can see it all. Deep down is a spirit that's still her. She's the same really, isn't she?"

Jackie leaves us, quietly moving to the cart to distribute medications. I feel my hands begin to shake.

I look at my mother. She's staring at the birds in the small cage across the room. Her rocker soothes her and her eyes close to slits. I take my thumb and trace her cheekbone. I rub the skin and watch it become young in my hands. The lines vanish, then reappear. Vanish, then reappear.

I remember being her young daughter, rubbing the rouge into her cheeks this way. She taught me how to find the bone and trace it. And then she placed the color on my finger and let me smooth it in. I could have stared at her forever. I still could.

My thumb moves softly from front to back, again and again. I watch the lines return and disappear. They will someday be the lines that already have begun to form across my own face.

I close my eyes. My mother's lines vanish altogether and all I feel is silk.

❧

Each day, the world is delivered to The Woods. Down the driveway trucks snort, winding slowly to their familiar destination. They turn a soft right by the pond and then back up to the delivery entrance, grunting into position in spurts of diesel. There boxes and boxes of supplies and food and medicines are unloaded.

They bring with them the services that residents once spent Saturday afternoons shopping for. They are Errands on Wheels. The trips to the grocery store, to the mall, to the pharmacy down the street are over. People here have given up their keys.

The only wheels people in Tanglewood see are wheels of carts full of juice and medicine and food trays, wheels of wheelchairs, wheels of X-ray machines, wheels of hospital gurneys.

The Blue Ribbon Meat truck arrives, advertising "New Food Traditions." Home Medical Service is perfect white, without a bruise. Spring Water Systems delivers Utah and Colorado to the door. Superior Dairy carries inside the farms that many of the people in The Woods once worked, brings cows and milk and cheese and memories of sweet green grass.

Residents here have tuned in nonstop to the country's biggest Home Shopping Channel.

CHAPTER FIVE

❧

Services

*I think all the people confined in the ward where
my friend Harry now is resident have gone beyond the
line. The line is incomprehensible to them certainly,
and they are unaware of having crossed the line. But
from the other side it is evident. The workers in the
place know it simply as a reality. Their care grows
more intense as the line grows more and more evident.*
ROBERT E. GARD, *Beyond the Thin Line*

·1·

My mother has guardian angels who help her from morning until night. When she awakens, an attendant
dresses her. She cannot, and would not, ever dress herself. Annabelle, who once sewed her way to fame, does not
understand fashion any longer and frequently resists the idea of
sleeves and buttons and clean underwear. She prefers just skin. In
early morning, her room becomes a battle zone.

At breakfast, the fight continues. If she gets up too early, she
hurries into the dining room and pilfers every place setting from

the tables. She must be watched and guarded until other residents appear—reinforcements, new troops—to protect their cups and saucers from her grand assault.

She cannot cut her food, so another attendant flutters to her side with a silver knife. Annabelle refuses to be fed and insists on eating with her fingers most of the time. She loves Froot Loops with milk, and eggs and toast. The staff works to let her eat at a table, but sometimes she wanders off eight or ten times at a meal and must be guided back, must be coaxed to the finish line.

Her medications throughout the day have to be disguised by the unit's magicians. Pills are crushed into soft, sweet foods. Syrups and powders are poured into flavored juices. Annabelle will no longer eat things that don't taste good.

At night, her clothes are as hard to remove as they were to put on earlier in the day. By 9:00 P.M., it seems to my mother that they have become a part of her, they are hers, and she hates to give them up. Sometimes her fight is so successful that her guardian angels let her sleep in polyester, in blouses with autumn leaves and pants with elastic waists.

They wait until morning and try again.

·2·

A plastic bulletin board rests at an angle on the six-foot fish tank that divides the living room. Permanent words in black form a banner at the top: "Today's Menu." Identical pictures of cornucopia decorate the top corners of the menu board. Underneath, other words linger for only one day in washable black marker.

BREAKFAST
Eggs or Malt-O-Meal

LUNCH
Chicken and Pasta

DINNER
Hawaiian Ham and Yams

Most of the people in Tanglewood cannot read the board, but they still like knowing that it's there. They know it means they will eat. They cannot read the words, but the words still make their stomachs growl. "When's lunch?" "When's supper?" The questions are asked over and over in Tanglewood, sometimes five minutes after a meal has been served.

People in Tanglewood cannot remember when they have eaten last. So they are always hungry. Except, of course, for those few in the rapidly progressive days of the final stage who have forgotten both hunger and thirst.

But most sit in chairs and dream of the next meal, of their favorite foods and drinks and desserts—especially of desserts, puddings and Jello and birthday cakes with butter icing.

"Where's my café au lait!" Kathleen mumbles, half asleep after a heavy lunch. "Turn around and make me some!" she orders the first person who comes into her sleepy view.

She remembers strolling out of her apartment to the coffee shop around the corner from her house and being drawn inside by the powerful odor of hazelnut beans. She remembers pouring rich cream and spooning sugar into coffee cups, and cannot get enough of it.

Never, never enough of it.

· 3 ·

My mother has pure blond hair. Pure gold. It never changed color from her girlhood. It never lost its thickness, or its strength.

Her first two years in Tanglewood, my mother eagerly accompanied an aide every Tuesday at 9:00 A.M. to the beauty shop. She sat still while the beautician washed her hair, rolled it in curlers, dried it, and combed it out. She recognized herself in the mirror and might have thought the woman busy behind her was Maxine.

Maxine had been my mother's beautician, and friend, for thirty years. Annabelle walked a mile every Saturday morning for her 9:00 A.M. appointment at Maxine's. Even after my father started taking her, and my mother sometimes wondered where she was going, the Saturday morning ritual continued. My mother never did her own hair. For her, going to Maxine's was going to heaven.

The memory of beauty shops and fingers tingling her scalp and simple conversations with women, just women, stuck with my mother a long, long time, and she would cooperate with the people in Tanglewood who helped prolong it. But during her third year there, she began to forget how good things felt.

I started to notice that sometimes her hair was very oily when I arrived, unset, unkempt. She would go to the shop only on a good day. She resisted and began to fear the small room down the hall from Tanglewood where the beautician in bubblegum pink waited for her.

She would no longer do these strange things that were asked of her. She would not wear a plastic cape that strangled her with Velcro, twist her neck into the lip of a porcelain shampoo bowl, tolerate painful plastic tubes that sometimes snapped her hair from her scalp, grill her head under a hot space capsule "for thirty minutes on high." When the aide came for her, she went screaming down the hall. If the screams didn't work, she would sit on the carpet and refuse to move. She would have to be carried, hospital-style, back into the unit.

For the first six months of her third year, I encouraged the staff to continue the trips to the beauty shop. But then I stopped her appointments. This would be the first time since 1928 that my mother would not have someone love her hair once a week, and I hated to have it end.

I stopped the appointments the day after I cut off her hair. I had found her sitting in a chair holding her hair back off her face with both hands. She was so enraged that she would not even look at me. She was holding both sides in tight clumps, determined to keep long, loose strands, delinquent curls, from slipping into her eyes. It was hard enough to see clearly anymore without this.

Her hair had become a horrible enemy. Even it seemed now

beyond her control. Her most glorious feature, the envy of other women all her life, the dream hair of every beautician, was attacking her.

I stepped to the nurse's station and asked to borrow a scissors. And then I asked an aide to help hold Annabelle's hands. While she did, I snipped my mother's long curls from her head. I cut close to her scalp, throwing lengths and lengths of hair recklessly onto the floor. Tons of it. I gave her something between a pixie and a shag. I gave her the worst haircut of her life.

It was just what she had wanted. After it was over, she smiled and went to sleep, and never looked exactly like Annabelle Coyne again.

·4·

When I arrive on Wednesday mornings, my mother smells like violets. She has just had her bath. Every Wednesday morning, when she's drowsy, only beginning to wake up, an aide steers my mother toward the bathing room and cleans her. This is the best time.

Today it is Wednesday, July 20, 1994. Exactly twenty-five years ago, Apollo 11 took the Eagle to the moon. Twenty-five years ago, an American flag was planted on Tranquility Base. Already the TV glows in the living area of Tanglewood. It's a day for celebration, even here.

Announcers are busy broadcasting news about the event on nearly every channel. Neil Armstrong is interviewed. So are residents from his hometown of Wapakoneta, Ohio. We hear the moon described again as having "a stark beauty all its own." A tape is played of the words that would lodge themselves in the memories of all Americans: "One small step for man, one giant leap for mankind." It has become the most famous slogan in the world.

In the bathing room, my mother is undressed and guided to a white plastic seat. She is strapped into the chair, secured with a seat belt. Slowly, the aide pushes a silver foot pedal at the base of

45

the tub and a hydraulic mechanism begins to lift my mother into the air, in loud clanks and spurts.

The television sends its signal down the hall. The names of Armstrong, Edwin Aldrin, and Michael Collins leave the lips of commentators. Statistics are cited with a sense of importance. Astronauts wore $100,000 moon suits. The trip to the moon was 240,000 miles. "All engines running. Lift-off!" shouts the voice of Launch Control over the TV.

My mother floats upward two feet and then is lowered into the full tub when the second pedal is pressed. A whoosh of decompression accompanies her landing in warm water. Her hair is washed with a movable spray. Water jets out from the sides to clean her lower body. Sometimes she splashes angrily. Other times she remembers the ritual of Saturday night baths on Evergreen Avenue, and drifts.

She presses her feet firmly into porcelain. She leaves her mark.

She is lifted into the air once again, lowered, and dried. Her mouth is cleaned. She is weighed and measured to make sure she has returned safely from her trip.

She has not gone far today, but she has traveled to the moon. She lives on the moon. She is the Woman in the Moon. Sometimes she flies beyond the moon, to a place no astronaut has ever been. She sees a crescent earth.

I lean close to her wet hair, closer to her lips, hoping for a slogan that will unite us. But on yet another Wednesday, my mother cannot give me this simple thing.

·5·

I find my mother outside in the patio sitting on the cement sidewalk, scooting restlessly toward her destiny. I wait for her to rise into my arms.

She is warm and I aim her toward the doors and air-conditioned coolness. She goes with me and chooses a geriatric chair by the supply closet to sit in. After I find a straight chair and move it beside her, I sit and fan her with the tablet in my purse.

I wish the breeze could stir words from her mouth, onto the page. I fan harder.

I watch her take her fingers and push them through her hair again and again, closing her eyes each time she sets her fingertips in place at her temples.

This is my cue. I reach into my purse a second time and remove a large pink comb. I begin to work the teeth across her scalp, over and over, front to back. She nestles close to me like a cat and bends her head so that the back can be done. I then travel to the other side.

Somewhere in my mother's brain, it is Saturday morning. Maxine is in the room.

The other women begin to gather around us.

"You can do mine if you want," Florence says, emerging from nowhere.

"Do you want to comb my hair too?" someone else calls out who wanders by.

"Do mine next. But be careful. I'm scared stiff," a third woman offers in mysterious code. "Where's your station?"

Five, ten versions of the same passion for combs and hair construct the path of my meditations as I lift my mother's short golden strands as high as they will go.

·6·

"Let's see your nails, Mrs. Blackburn," a morning aide gently orders. She will make the same request of every resident in the room, checking for breaks, rough edges, tears in cuticles.

"Nice," she says to Mrs. Blackburn. "Yours are always nice." Mrs. Blackburn, from New York City, loves the compliment. She is proud of her appearance in a way few others here can be. She stares at pictures of herself on the bulletin board and smiles. She has been named Resident of the Week. She is the only woman who can paint her own nails, keeping to the boundaries. She is the only woman who wears jewelry and never seems to lose it, or have it lost. She wears pearl earrings that weigh down her lobes, a sparkling blue bracelet made of aquamarines, and a cameo always pinned to her fur piece. "It was made in Italy from conch shells," she tells me whenever I admire it. Mrs. Blackburn is elegant. She is from another world.

But most women in Tanglewood are not like her and secretly want the aide to find something wrong, take them by the hand, and sit them at the table for a manicure.

A paisley bag soon appears from the supply room. Nail files, emery boards, scissors, and bottles of nail polish line up on the table. Old women close their eyes and wait for the small sounds of nails being shaped and pointed, for the strong smell of Maybelline and Revlon. They wait for the aide to blow her warm breath fast across the new color. They wait for something special to happen because they have had their nails done today.

My mother does not cooperate on cue any longer. So I have become her manicurist as well as her beautician. I carry a small scissors, a nail file, a toenail clipper, a razor, tweezers, and nail polish in my purse at all times. I scrape my mother's chin free of ancient women's hairs, tweeze an eyebrow, clip and file fingernails and toenails when she's still.

I don't know why I worry about nails any longer. I guess I think that maybe, just once more, my mother will notice the shimmering color, understand its meaning, and remember warm summer nights.

I just want her to be ready when the carriage pulls up to the door.

CHAPTER SIX

∾

Work

As a child Cora had watched him fixing radios or
fishing, deft and definite in his movements, his gaze
glazed in concentration, absorbed in his activity—
enslaved to something at its center.

CARRIE FISHER, *Delusions of Grandma*

·1·

Helen distributes the bibs. Helen lives to distribute the bibs. She waits nervously, with great anticipation, for 11:30 A.M. and 5:00 P.M. These are the times when she's permitted to go into the linen closet and collect twenty-four blue bibs with Velcro tabs. By then, the residents have all been positioned in their seats. Helen winds a blue bib sensuously around each neck and makes sure it's secure.

Sometimes the staff grows annoyed with Helen's obsession with the bibs. She frequently cannot concentrate on her own lunch or dinner because she knows her job is not yet finished. After dessert and coffee, Helen is permitted to remove the bibs and place them in the dirty linen container down the hall from the dining area.

Helen often rises impatiently from her seat and begins removing the bibs too soon.

"And how was your food?" she'll kindly ask as she rips a bib from around a neck.

"Sit down for a few minutes, Helen! Chill!" an aide shouts. "Let them eat in peace for a change."

Helen sits when she is commanded but will forget the order within thirty seconds. She will rise again and renew her attack on the dirty blue bibs.

The staff may correct her once more, but maybe not. Every meal is Helen's party. They let her play the part she has rehearsed all her life.

·2·

Gene must have had patio furniture.

Whenever the wind blows a little harder than usual, or rain begins to fall, or sometimes just at the end of a day, Gene hurries to the patio and starts his routine. He's very slow and his muscles are weak, but one by one he lifts the chairs and arranges them on top of the umbrella table. He knows the pattern.

By carefully folding the chairs into one another and building two tiers, he manages to place all eight under the protection of canvas. They are all safe on top of the table, with only an occasional inch or two of metal frame hanging from the edge.

Gene has long ago forgotten his wife and his children, his brothers and his sisters. But he has not forgotten this job that needs to be done in bad weather.

·3·

Louie is a large woman with the prettiest smile in the unit. She always wears yellow. Yellow polyester blouses, yellow running pants. And when her daughters visit, they visit in yellow. Louie spends her days being a young mother again. She fusses with the other residents and gossips.

She makes bandages out of newspaper and head compresses out of underwear in her drawer. She heals people all day.

Under her arm are her constant companions—a large fur monkey and a Dalmatian puppy. She dresses them, combs them, feeds them. You'll see her sit for hours talking to her synthetic children, sometimes tears welling in her eyes from a mother's deep disappointment or concern.

Louie exhausts herself in affection. Her work has no end. Sometimes she'll fall asleep with her forehead balanced strangely on the edge of a hard table. Her own comfort never seems to be an issue.

She never complains.

·4·

Work is what everyone who ever knew my mother remembers about her, along with her spectacular blond hair. She started working at the age of fourteen for a grocer in downtown Akron, and never stopped. As one of the older children in a poor family of seven, with an alcoholic father, she had no choice. Work got in her veins. After school, after work at the grocery store, she went home to clean the coal stove or help her mother, Anna, make the bread-and-butter pickles she was famous for in the neighborhood, in "Goosetown" where the German immigrants settled in Akron, Ohio.

She knew instinctively that work was better for her than alcohol. A million times better. She showed me every day of her life that nothing is as true and permanent and liberating as work. Nothing. Absolutely nothing. It was her salvation. It was her freedom. It was the only thing she had that was her own.

·5·

Three years ago, my mother could help the staff set the table. And then, after she forgot what forks and spoons were for, Esther let her sweep the linoleum area of the floor. She would sweep all afternoon, into the evening, until someone took the broom away.

Now, Esther pretends she does not see my mother remove the clear plastic that wraps the cushions on the living room chairs. Of course the plastic must be replaced every time my mother rips it off—too many residents have long ago lost control of bladders and bowels. But Esther knows my mother loves to work. She knows this is the best that Annabelle can do.

·6·

My mother is happy today. She smiles. She plays with my hair. She takes my hand and directs me to the patio doors. We exit the unit and go outside.

The patio is the size of a good garden in the suburbs. A small green is in the center, with an umbrella table, the eight chairs entrusted to Gene, two medium-sized maple trees, and a charcoal grill. A cement walkway surrounds the green. To the right of the walkway is a three-foot border of flowering bushes and wooden planters with annuals exclusively in purple: petunias, pansies, impatiens. On the north side of the patio is a fence dotted with window boxes. On the west side, the landscape crew plants a few tomatoes each year.

We circle the patio, and my mother shakes her head at the bench (I do not know what complaint she is trying to register). She admires the petunias, touching several in a huge wooden box. But she soon loses interest. After the petunias, she seems to forget the plants and notice nothing. She stares ahead of her, stoop-shouldered, fierce, bothered by a maple leaf that brushes her forehead. She pulls me hard.

She is glad when I open the door to Tanglewood. She steps inside, relieved to be in a simpler place.

·7·

Two years ago, Annabelle spent hours on the patio every warm day of the year. She would assemble curious bouquets of flowers, made of maple leaves and rhododendron blossoms, of clover and impatiens blooms. Gradually, she would forget how to distinguish flowers from weeds, stems from blossoms, vegetables from stones. She would uproot annuals. One late summer she proudly presented Esther with a skirtful of green tomatoes. She had picked every single one. They never ripened, even placed on the warmest window sills.

But now the patio is too mysterious for her. She has forgotten what the soil means. Colored leaves that mat the ground in fall frighten her when they break in her hands.

The surprise of spring will never return.

·8·

After my mother retired, the grass, the bushes, the small flower garden around her birdbath became her obsession. Became her new work. The privet hedge that divided my parents' property from the neighbors' was perfectly trimmed. My mother would look with worry at my dad when he jammed an oily baseball cap on his head, draped his heavy hedge trimmer over his shoulder like a logger, and took off for the privet hedge. She would follow him and with her fingers remove *every* leaf, *every* cutting, that fell onto the yard or drive. She would snip away my father's errors with a scissors.

She would edge the sidewalks with the same scissors, hundreds of feet of sidewalk. Painful blisters on her hands would turn to callouses by June.

In the early spring, she would rip out poison ivy from the back bushes with her bare hands, never affected by its poison, never even knowing it was a hazardous plant until I told her.

She would plant common annuals in the two-foot ring around the birdbath. Marigolds, snapdragons, petunias bloomed throughout the summer, and she would stare at them through the window by the kitchen sink, hands wrinkled with detergent, rings resting in an imitation Wedgwood dish.

She would worry about the flowers and scold my father gently when he mowed too close to her border.

There was not a single dandelion in their entire yard.

In the late '80s, I began to plant the garden by the birdbath for my sick mother, and my son began to mow the grass for my ailing father. We became the Lawn and Garden Dream Team and roared into their drive with our tools every Wednesday afternoon of the next three summers.

·9·

Gene dresses like no one else in the unit. He wears a soft cotton shirt, a striped tie, a burnt sienna sweater, and a suit coat every day. No matter what the temperature is, Gene is dressed for the office.

On the walls of Gene's room are certificates of dentistry. Wrought iron bookshelves hold professional journals and heavy reference texts. He sits in his room sometimes in a comfortable chair. He never reads anymore. He just stares at his books, one hand always resting softly on the top of the collection.

Gene shuffles on his heels around the unit, quiet and happy. The toes of his black leather shoes seem empty and stick up in the air like clown shoes. Often you can find him in front of the oversized clock that hangs on the wall opposite the nurse's station, a huge thing two feet by two feet with enormous hands. He stands fiddling awkwardly with the stem of his own watch, trying hard to set the time. He looks up at the clock on the wall, then down at his wrist. Up then down, again and again. But the task always proves too difficult. Gene shakes his head and shuffles to the next room with the stem of his watch still loose.

I see him worry when he faces toothless residents. He drops his head and looks with concern over the rim of his wire glasses. He starts to point at pink gums, but has nothing to say, and walks away.

At the end of every meal, he picks his spectacular teeth.

·10·

"It's a family heir-doom," Gloria tells me. I've just asked her about the cane she always carries, with a mysterious gold ring right below the hook of the handle, like a cigar band.

" '30," she reads the gold, following my stare. "That's the year I graduated. My parents were married in 1900. It was my Uncle Paul's walking stick, made from shark bones, and now it's mine. Who would have believed it!"

Gloria smiles broadly, revealing no teeth, just an enormous hole the size of a peach. She glances at the birds in the metal cage. "My job was to deliver the baby turkeys. When I was in the fifth and sixth grades, I carried them in my bare arms and walked from Grant to Market."

I tried to picture Market Street, to imagine its shops and businesses, to see the poultry farm that Gloria apparently had been hired to supply.

"I was just a little girl and I did that all by myself!"

Her speech shifts to its common refrain. "Did you ever see William Nevel? He's so handsome. Six foot two!"

"How long were you married, Gloria?"

"Oh it's still *brewing!*" she corrects me. "But he's down in the basement now with the other men. That's how it goes. Men group with men. Women group with women. But Bill and I are very much in love, although his interests are different from mine and we're separated by parties. We're very much in love."

Gloria looks at me. "Did you ever date the Nevel boys?" she wonders. "Do you live here or did you come in for the party?"

"I don't live here. I never dated the Nevel boys," I tell her.

I stroke my mother's cheek and let my thumb glide across her ear. Gloria watches, and smiles her peach smile once more in our direction.

"You're being remembered," she tells Annabelle.

Angie, the activity director, has come over to summon Gloria to the puzzle table. They are working on a jigsaw puzzle of a small white kitten and she is invited. Perky, Angie's green parakeet from home, is on her shoulder and chirps the invitation in Gloria's ear.

"Well, it was so nice to see you," she tells me. "*And* your escort," she adds, nodding toward my mother. "But he's so quiet," she comments, shaking her head.

"From Ivy to Grant to Market!" she shouts on her way to puzzles, waving Uncle Paul's cane victoriously in the air. "I carried baby birds all that way."

·11·

Annabelle was different from her sisters, from her friends, from the neighbor women all along her street. She was never a "home person" and she had the courage to face that truth about herself without the guilt of her generation. Maybe it had something to do with the way the stars lined up on September 5, 1910, the day of her birth. She was born on a Monday, the first Monday of September—on Labor Day. On the day she took her first breath, people across the nation were already picnicking in her honor.

Today 80 percent of women with children have full-time jobs. In the '40s, the figure was only 10 percent. My mother was one of them.

Within six months of a resignation prompted by my birth, she changed her mind and returned full-time to the Food Service division of the Akron Public Schools, once more keeping the books exact, to the penny, through her meticulous use of ledgers, adding machine, and a brain that was years ahead of her high school education, or even her rank as valedictorian of her high school class.

Sometimes when help was slim in the warehouses, she would spend her lunch hour aboard a forklift, scooping huge boxes full of giant cans of Campbell's tomato soup onto shelves.

Or if a cook was sick in a school, my mother would snap a hairnet onto her head and ladle bright yellow macaroni onto plastic plates.

She would remain with the Food Service Department, full-time, until her retirement in 1973.

In my jewelry box is a bracelet with links of sterling and a single circular silver charm. One side reads "Annabelle Coyne," the other, "Akron Public Schools 1928–73."

They were the happiest years of her life.

As you meander down the nursing wing on your way to Tanglewood, colorful birds in thin frames greet you on the walls. They are reproductions of Audubon prints. There are Baltimore Orioles and Brown Pelicans, Great Blue Herons and Wood Ducks.

But in the entranceway to Tanglewood, between the steel doors and the nurse's station, the motif suddenly changes, without warning.

Flowers line the walls now. Not just any flowers. Framed at three-foot intervals are illustrations of irises. No other flowers, only irises. They are mounted in heavy Victorian frames, labeled with their names in Latin and French at the bottom in delicate script. Iris Amana (Iris Agreable), Iris Zyphioides (Iris Faux-Xyphium), Iris Fimbriata (Iris Frangee).

They seem inappropriate at first. Huge, lush purple blossoms disturb their frames. The wood is ready to split at every corner seam. Petals fold in sensual curves. Iris Chrysographes, the Black Iris, quivers restlessly behind glass lined with fine cracks.

Irises force you to look at them. Even in Tanglewood.

CHAPTER SEVEN

❧

Love and Sex

Despite all my difficulties, I now felt like Libido Lady.
DIANA FRIEL McGOWIN, *Living in the Labyrinth*

·1·

My mother sits at one of the four-person dining room tables turning the pages of *Mirabella* magazine. She seems not to notice the pictures at first, but to be obsessed with turning each sheet, clean and separate, one at a time. When pages are caught together, she pries the corner with her thumbnail until the static releases them and they separate.

Midway through, she stops at a picture of three women, nude from the waist up, shoulders brushing and heads leaning toward the camera at odd angles. These are the new models for Bergdorf

Goodman, women as strange-looking as the three witches in *Macbeth.*

Annabelle tears the sheet from the magazine and gives it to me.

Millie, dressed in blue cotton, five round glimmering sequins dotting the low neckline of her made-in-India dress and a white Hanes undershirt sticking five inches above, watches my mother turn the pages and proudly rip the Bergdorf models from their spine. Millie grows excited, panting hard through her nose. She laughs.

"Tits!" Millie shouts as she points at the glossy sheet of paper.

·2·

Mr. Henry Wittner used to live in Tanglewood. Now he shares a double room in the nursing section with another man. But he gets lonely. He remembers better days down the hall.

When no one is looking, Henry sneaks from his room and pumps his wheelchair quickly in the direction of Tanglewood. He'll sit a minute, staring innocently, whistling a little, twiddling his thumbs, fooling a nurse or two who think he's just following his exercise program and pausing to catch his breath.

When the women in white disappear into rooms to dispense pills, into closets to arrange supplies, behind stations to call families and doctors, Mr. Wittner turns sharply to the left and races to Tanglewood, looking behind him like a guilty boy. Then he waits. And waits. Until, magically, some visitors exit and he asks them to please hold the door for him—he isn't quite strong enough, he tells them, just an old man. They smile and oblige.

Henry has won again. He braces the door with his chair. Then he quickly slicks his hair back with both hands, adjusts the half-eaten package of Fig Newtons stuck in his shirt pocket, sits up straight, checks his chin for crumbs, tightens his belt a notch, and completes his journey.

"Not you again, Henry," the nurse says in amusement. She pauses, seeing his disappointment. "Do you want to stay a little while?" she pampers him.

He smiles and rolls his chair into the living room. A movie is on, but he positions himself so that his back faces the TV screen and he faces the five women vaguely interested in the flicker of film in front of them.

"Well," he smiles, "I'm fit as a fiddle and I'm ready for love, ladies!"

No one notices him. They continue with their naps and half-interest in the old movie that promises a different kind of love than Henry's.

"Hey!" he says, more loudly. "Want a Fig Newton? I'm hot to trot!"

One woman takes her cane and pushes on the wheel of his chair. Mr. Henry Wittner doesn't seem to mind. He's a few inches farther away now, but it doesn't seem to matter. It doesn't change a thing.

· 3 ·

My mother is running her thumbnail across the seams of the vinyl tablecloth. She rises and moves to chairs occupied by afternoon sleepers, feeling armrests, slats, springs on rockers. I hold my breath and pray that no one moves, that her fingers are not pinched by someone's bad dream.

She roams to the other side of the room and once again takes off the plastic covers from the seat pillows. She finds a new chair in the area by the nurse's station and sits.

Next to the magazine table not far from us sits Isabelle, curiously annoyed with me, but I don't know why. She is a very polite woman, always smiling, always kind to my mother. Always telling me how beautiful Annabelle is, her pal. When she tells me I resemble my mother, it is a compliment. I light up. But today Isabelle is someone else.

"Are you CRAZY?!" she yells at me.

Jackie, who has taken the shift after Esther's, hears Isabelle, lifts her head over the counter, and tells me that Isabelle was an elementary school principal and often issues "helpful" instructions.

"I don't know sometimes, Isabelle," I answer. "Maybe I am."

"You're hardly wearing any clothes!" she whispers loudly. It's hot outside, ninety-five degrees. I have on blue jeans and a sleeveless top. No one in Tanglewood ever wears a sleeveless top, but I'd never noticed before.

"Put something on, for heaven's sake, child!" She points her index finger at me and shakes her head.

As senseless as it seems, I feel obscenely out of place for a moment. I have offended Isabelle and broken the rules of Tanglewood.

My mother, totally unaware of what has just taken place, rests her head on my bare shoulder. I feel better, though I don't know why, and stroke her hair.

·4·

Geraldo is gliding across the afternoon screen. In front of him are today's freaks: a fourteen-year-old girl, her thirty-four-year-old lover, and the girl's mother.

"But do you really think your daughter can know what love is at her age?" he asks the mother. The audience applauds his question and jeers at the trio.

"Sure," the mother says. "Love is love at any age. You look at him." She points at the rough character sitting beside her angry-looking daughter whose skirt has disappeared into the folds of her lap. "He loves my little girl. And she loves him. It's pretty simple."

A few residents of Tanglewood stare at the scene in front of them, but see nothing strange. They yawn. Occasionally they turn and watch sunlight pour through the west window.

·5·

Benny is a little man. A cute man. He's so thin that no pants stay up without the help of his bowling suspenders. He was on a league most of his adult life. His trophies line his dresser. Someone who loved him must have found him the wonderful suspenders he constantly wears, suspenders with black bowling balls and gleaming white pins scattered up and down red elastic.

He has boyish brown eyes, a sly smile, and a complexion dotted by both age spots and freckles. He is gap-toothed and large-eared. Benny looks a little like a rabbit if you come upon him suddenly.

It is clear that Benny must have spent his life loving women. Or trying to. Even though now he grows annoyed very quickly with flirtations he initiates (typically within thirty seconds he's telling a woman he's just propositioned to go to hell), that doesn't stop him from looking for love in Tanglewood.

When you see Benny, he most likely will be holding the hand of a female resident, or of an indulgent staff member or a nurse. He loves to hold hands and kiss them. It's his occupation now.

One day after Benny kissed my hand, he began singing. He stared at me with filmy eyes and broke into a beautiful tenor voice. He sang the Kyrie, remembering the Catholic mass, perhaps having been the cantor for his parish. His past swelled up into his throat, into sound, and his eyes reddened. "Kyrie eleison." *Lord, have mercy on us.* "Christe eleison." *Christ, have mercy on us.* Over and over. *Lord, have mercy.*

He stopped suddenly and stared at his small slippered feet. Then his head snapped up rapidly.

"SEX!"

And then, "Will you do that?"

I tried to convince myself that he couldn't possibly be putting the two thoughts together. I issued my typical response to the inarticulate mutterings of Tanglewood residents, a response that generally brought reassurance. "Maybe," I nodded.

"Maybe?" he repeated. "MAYBE!" He dropped my hand violently, shook his head, muttered "Ah, shit" under his breath, turned, and began to prowl the streets once more.

·6·

Benny's new rival is Bob, a man from Canada who recently entered the unit. Bob has fallen in love with Louie.

He sits beside her, holding her hand and looking into her

65

sleepy face through glasses so thick they make his eyes look like giant shooter marbles. He wants to walk. And he wants to walk with this woman in yellow.

With great difficulty, Bob rises and stands in front of Louie. She does not respond, except to allow her limp arm to travel with his hand. "Come on. Let's go. You want to walk with me?"

Louie says nothing, drifting in and out of an afternoon nap, tired after a day full of nothing but labors of love. She is loved out for now. Bob's words are only background music.

"Say something," he begs. His voice is loud and Louie snaps awake. She leans forward and begins to fix his collar, play with the buttons on his shirt, twirl his chest hair around her finger.

"I love you," he says as he bends over and kisses her on the lips. "You're a nice girl. I don't care what they say. Come on," he pleads once more, pulling her toward him.

Benny sees the kiss and moves quickly in its direction.

"Goddamn!" he swears angrily at Bob, a man twice his size. "Honey, honey," he says softly to Louie.

"Do you know what the nice girl's called?" Bob asks Benny, unaware of Benny's jealousy. "Talk to me!" he screams in her direction.

Benny knows from the force of the sound that he cannot win here and backs away. He unzips his pants and pees a warm yellow puddle on the linoleum, marking his territory. "Goddamn. Jesus Christ," he mumbles, swatting his hand in disgust.

Bob too knows he cannot win, not his way. He sits down again and places his cane vertically between his chair and Louie's. Louie smiles, used to having her own way with men, and they cup their hands together on the top of Bob's cane and kiss on the lips once more.

·7·

Kathleen spots me holding a cup of cranapple juice that an aide has just poured for Annabelle. She lifts herself from her seat and comes over to say hello, to me, to the juice. She is always thirsty.

"What a pretty color!" she says, peering into the cup. "It would make wonderful jewelry. And I have plenty of that!"

She thinks about what she has said, examining her fingers and her wrists. "Well," Kathleen corrects herself. "I used to. Now I just have these." She wiggles the plastic hospital band on her left wrist that displays her name, her social security number, information about her doctor. She rubs the engraving on the silver ID bracelet that circles her right wrist: "Memory Impaired."

I look at the small rubies on my wedding band and present them to her for approval, for comfort. "These are the color of cranberries, Kathleen," I say.

Forgetting the subject of color, Kathleen smiles slyly. "When is *that* going to be active?" she asks, pointing to the stones.

I'm confused and say the only thing I can: "I don't know."

"Well," she advises, "you're wise to wait. That's something you want to be darn sure about."

She thinks I'm engaged. The ring is a promise.

Kathleen strolls back toward her seat, but then remembers something and heads full speed in my direction, breathing hard by the time she arrives.

"Listen," she says. "Try to pick a doctor if you can."

"Thanks," I tell her.

She winks and hurries back once more to her seat, this time with a mission. The juice cart has arrived and she wants to order cranapple. And rubies and diamonds and surgeons, and everything she sees in the sparkling drops that fill her cup.

·8·

Gloria is sitting outside on the patio, dressed again today as green as the grass below her feet. From behind her Gene approaches, shuffling and stooped. He has a broken petunia in his hand that was just picked and discarded by some other lost resident.

"Want a flower?" he shyly asks Gloria.

She can't believe this gift. "Thank you so much!" she cries. "Imagine sending me a flower!" She spreads her fingers wide and pounds her hand against her chest.

Gene has turned to enter Tanglewood.

"Where is he?" she asks, worried. "I have to tell him. Isn't that lovely of him?" She rises slowly, painfully, but spots him by the door.

"Thank you!" she yells, now moving twice his speed. "I want to shake your hand," she says, catching him. And she does.

She puts her arm through his and they enter the unit together. "Have you had much snow?" she asks him, and then quickly shakes her head. "No, much ice, I mean." She knows this too is not right. "Much sunshine?" She has it now.

Gloria strolls by the game table. "They're all busy playing. I have to tell the family I'm home. Walking is a little hard."

She finds the nurse's station and proudly shows them her petunia. "Isn't this wonderful?" she asks. Pointing to Gene, she adds, "My nephew gave it to me."

"No!" Gene counters. "I'm not—"

But it doesn't matter. They walk arm in arm to an empty table and continue praising petunias and men who present them so gallantly to lovers, to aunts.

·9·

For two years after my mother entered Tanglewood, my husband courted her. Every week, on Saturday, he would arrive to take her out for peach pie a la mode.

She had no idea who he was, exactly, but every idea that he was hers. "He's *mine!*" she'd announce to everyone within hearing distance when he came to fetch her. Something inside still remembered the chicken he barbecued so many times on the grill, just for her. And the corn he rolled lovingly onto her plate, dripping in sweet butter.

They'd walk hand in hand to the car for the short ride down

the street to pie. For part of their courtship, she still carried a purse.

The restaurant owners and servers were waiting for them. My husband and Annabelle were an item.

People who worked at the restaurant loved my mother and understood her habits. They knew she must be seated and served immediately. They knew that she would become suspicious and worried if her food, for any reason, came out of the kitchen late.

As her disease grew worse, they cut her pie for her and gave her extra silverware, extra napkins. They were not surprised if she scooped tip money from the previous order into her pocket, or the vanilla ice cream that topped her pie onto the floor. They said nothing when she stole packets of Sweet 'N Low and stuffed them in her Cobbies. She was theirs, and that was all they cared about.

And then one day my husband realized there could be no more outings to the restaurant for peach pie. The courtship phase of my mother's disease had ended. She was fighting seat belts, opening car doors in the middle of highways, losing her appetite for even her favorites—peach pie and my husband.

From now on, any dessert we would eat with my mother would have to be on her terms, and on her turf, not ours.

·10·

Florence still gets her hair permed every three months in the beauty shop. She uses a walker but enjoys most just sitting in her room, alone. She has beautiful mahogany furniture from her past, a television and radio of her own, mirrors, plants, a Turkish rug. Frequently she patrols the halls. She stands at the edge of her room and casts judgment.

She doesn't like my mother. When my mother babbles toothlessly at her or drifts into her room, she lifts her walker and pokes my mother in the side. Florence is afraid of what has happened to Annabelle.

One day Florence seemed especially angry. She was watching

the parade of residents in front of her room, people drifting nowhere or wanting a look outside or hoping to find the home they remembered that was better than this one. She watched the large, waistless bodies glide past her, the colorful sweat suits, the tennis shoes, the canes, the walkers, the wheelchairs, the ancient heads with short gray hair, or none.

"You can't tell men from women in this goddamn place," she scowled. She pointed directly at my mother with the rubber tips of her walker. "That woman looks like Abraham Lincoln!"

Florence squeezed her new beauty-shop curls and disappeared inside.

·11·

I arrive to the key of E, to the unexpected sound of Mendelssohn's Wedding March from *A Midsummer Night's Dream*. At 2:31 P.M., on the upstroke of the clock, the bride and groom begin their walk down the sacred aisle between the rows of chairs in Tanglewood toward the altar where they will be married.

Angie, the activity director, has planned a mock wedding for the residents. Actually, the event began a week before with a bridal shower, and then a fashion show on the patio that featured discarded evening gowns and wedding apparel from the closets of aides and nurses.

The bride is a young aide who really will be married in October. Her groom couldn't come to Tanglewood this afternoon, so she has brought her brother. He is tall enough. A little young, perhaps, but no one minds.

The room is glorious. It has been transformed by donations of flowers from local florists. One arrangement includes huge irises, purple tulips, baby's breath, and peach roses. An altar has been constructed from a juice cart draped with a hospital sheet. On top are wild flowers, purple spiderwort and daisies that Angie plucked from the road on her way into work. On each resident's chair a purple or pink balloon is tied. A sheet cake made that

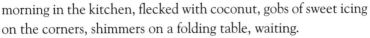

morning in the kitchen, flecked with coconut, gobs of sweet icing on the corners, shimmers on a folding table, waiting.

Everyone is dressed up, including the nurses and aides. My mother, asleep, wears a suit. Nylons gleam up and down the rows, and men have on leather shoes.

The bride marches down the aisle on the arm of Mr. Miller. It seems correct that he should have this honor, for today is Mr. Miller's birthday. He's seventy-five and his wife has ordered a cake from the local bakery with purple roses and the words "To My Husband." Today is a two-cake occasion.

Behind the bride is the flower girl dressed in lime chiffon, tilting awkwardly in her first pair of white heels. She is the daughter of a Tanglewood nurse.

Mr. Miller gives the bride away and she faces the priest behind the altar, Mr. Simmons from assisted living. He has dressed in a choir robe and collar this afternoon to marry the couple. The groom walks to his bride's side and takes her hand. "Beautiful, so beautiful!" Gloria cries. Gene claps, unable to contain his joy. His perfect teeth send white light into the room.

"Dearly beloved," Mr. Simmons begins, reading from a blue manila folder he has carefully prepared for the occasion, "we are gathered here today to join this man and this woman in holy matrimony." The service continues, and ends with a kiss. There is no embarrassment between the bride and her brother. They kiss sweetly, as real lovers would.

For several minutes after bouquets are thrown in the air, wedding pictures are taken. Residents are encouraged to stand alongside the bride and groom and smile. Gloria wants to be first. "She's just a neighbor," Gloria tells everyone, looking at the bride and squeezing her tightly around her slim waist. "But a very good neighbor," she adds.

Angie tries to get Gloria to kiss the bride's cheek, but Gloria is confused and can't understand the request that's being made of her. She tilts her head, changes position, tries to cooperate in new ways. Finally, she understands and kisses the bride. "You are practicing on me for the real thing!" she teases, nudging the couple.

Someone changes the music in the tape deck to Lawrence Welk Champagne tunes. The flower girl distributes napkins and forks from a ribboned basket while the activity director cuts the cake and places large slices on paper plates. These too are handed to residents. My mother still sleeps, so I take a piece and hold it for her.

Gloria is amazed by all of it. She loves her cake and she loves this wedding. "I can't believe all this has happened today!" she exclaims.

After the cake is gone and the crumbs licked clean from plates, the dancing is ready to begin. Someone removes Lawrence Welk from the tape deck and inserts Polka's Greatest Hits.

"It's time for the bride and groom to dance, don't you think? We'll clap and get them up here!" Angie sets the rhythm and hands begin to join hers, calling for the dance.

I hear the bride whisper words to her brother about how to do a polka two-step. He smiles, stumbles a little, but bounces with energy up and down the aisle. Then, the bride and the groom ask residents to dance. And they do. They love it. They love these two young people already.

Gloria dances in the groom's arms. The "Somewhere My Love Polka" is playing loudly in the background. The groom is nearly six feet tall. "You dance like my husband," she tells him. "Let me kiss your cheek." She lifts her lips and finds his young face.

Kathleen is exhausted by her dance with the bride and sits down. "This reminds me of my own wedding," she says, "although I don't remember being quite this tired. I was married in Uncle Howard's house on Woodlawn Avenue."

The bride and groom must leave now. Residents understand they must give them up to the honeymoon. The couple parades once more, stopping briefly to shake hands with each guest, and kiss them.

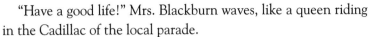

"Have a good life!" Mrs. Blackburn waves, like a queen riding in the Cadillac of the local parade.

"Keep yourself fresh with that veil!" Gloria advises the bride.

"I wish you well. I really do," Gene offers through his tears.

Gloria has one more thing to say before the couple departs. "The most important thing is love! Love! Do you hear me! *Love!*" She points her cane high in the air.

My mother has finally opened her eyes, awakened by Gloria's words. I press the frosting to her mouth and she tastes it. She focuses on the plate and breaks off a large piece of cake, moving it to her lips, eager for this snack.

The piece is too much for a single bite. But when she's chewed the first, and ready to squeeze the rest into her mouth, she sees me and stops. Like a bride, or a groom, she feeds me cake and icing with her fingers. My lips fold around pure sugar and flesh.

Tanglewood is bordered on three sides by a dense woods.
Every window in the unit faces north or south or west,
and every view offers a glimpse of wild flowers, black
trunks, and knotted shrubs and bushes. East windows ex-
posing cars, the street, and civilization are absent here.

Country living and rustic peace are advertised in the
literature for The Woods.

But the rich border of forest around the complex is too
disturbing. There are no cows, no quiet streams, no
soothing waterfalls, no peaceful pastures. There are no
bowers or trellises, no pretty garden spots.

The trees are too high here. Phlox, blackberries, wild
roses, Queen Anne's lace, thistles edge the woods. Then,
bushes with strange triangular clusters of furry burnt orange flowers that point straight up begin to appear, and
small maples and mountain ash. Behind it all are thick-
trunked trees, monsters that block the sun and darken the
rooms of residents.

It is untamed land, wild, full of weird whispers and
strange sounds from the earth and the wind.

Sometimes, landscapers are hired to whack away large
branches from trees. If left alone, limbs begin to crawl
and creep through the slats of the white patio fence. The
woods want to come inside.

CHAPTER EIGHT

Paranoia

They found her in the farthest pasture.
Tugging feebly at her print dress caught
in a tangle of barbed wire, she stood
with wide eyes, watching the Indians
come from behind the trees.

BETTIE SELLERS,
"All on a Summer's Afternoon,"

·1·

The woman in green sits with the nursing staff at shift change. Each shift informs the next about the daily status of every resident and discusses any problems. Gloria is nearly screaming, but no one says much. Occasionally someone leans over to rub her hands, both of which tightly brace the arms of her chair. But her loud statements and occasional screams bother no one.

"There's a red light!" she yells, pointing to something others cannot see. "Oh my God! Please call for help!"

An aide smiles at Gloria and laughs softly. "It's all right, Gloria. Nothing's wrong."

"There's a red light, and nothing's wrong? You just laugh it off?"

Around the corner, a television, volume low, plays *Curse II: The Bite*. Someone has forgotten to monitor the program. A cheap horror movie with Jill Schoelen and J. Eddie Peck sneaks onto the screen. It's about young lovers who go through an old desert nuclear test-site full of mutant snakes.

"The red light! Somebody please, please, do something. It may be too late. Look in front of you!"

I glance around the corner and see police cars, lights spinning on top of roofs, heading toward the rescue of the young woman, now stuck in vile quicksand with monster snakes. An officer throws a rope to the woman, beautiful even slathered with mud. The snake lifts its head, ready to devour its prey, but is shot to pieces by the woman's rescuer. Bits of the mutated beast fly across the screen. The woman is safe.

By the time I turn my attention back to Gloria, she has forgotten the danger she was in. I wave to her across the room, and smile with amusement and relief.

"Hi!" she shouts. "You always bring me so much good luck!"

I have no idea what she is talking about.

· 2 ·

Every fall, my parents took a trip to Exchange, West Virginia, to visit cousins. At the end of the summer of 1987, as at the end of other summers, I asked my father when they would be leaving. He said they were not going this year, maybe never again. Something had happened last time, something horrible.

"Last October," my father began. He swallowed hard and started over. "Last October Mother ran out of the house screaming, down the dirt road, up into the hills. We all hunted for her. It took us two hours to find her. It was terrible. Terrible."

What was in your head, Mother, as you screamed your way

higher and higher up the mountain? I heard you scream once. Remember? I was a little girl. It was snowing and the window shade shivered back and forth from the air seeping through the cracks. I thought it was the wind at first, that screaming. I wanted it to be. I listened and waited. And then, finally, far too late, I remembered you. You had gone outside with the garbage from dinner in your hand, coatless, and had not returned. I pulled the door hard, causing a row of bells on a red plastic ribbon to break into alarm. And there you were stretched out on the icy drive, arm tucked under your breast and neck like the wing of a crippled bird. But the pain was so horrible, the arm so shattered, that you couldn't stop screaming even for my sake, even for a daughter only eight who wanted you to stop.

And did you stop when they found you on the hill? Or was your wait too long again? Was the pain still there even when old faces found you in the moonlight?

·3·

Shortly after their fall trip was canceled, I began noticing that my mother looked at me with suspicion. I had never seen it on her face before. It was not a part of her nature. Ever. She would join my father and me in the living room of their house on Sunday afternoons, as she always had done, but now would stay only a few minutes. She would listen to us talk and begin to suspect something we could not even imagine. She would flick her fingernails on the fabric of the chair and shift her eyes from one corner of the room to the other as if they were following some ominous pendulum visible only to her. Her fingers would move rapidly up and down her clothing, picking, bunching, clawing at things that were not there.

She would rise and hurry to the kitchen for a glass of water from the sink, talking to herself loudly. She would scramble down the cellar stairs to sort through clothes, hurry to the upstairs bathroom, and then across to her bedroom. We would hear her slam the door.

My father would shake his head, place his elbows on his knees, and cup his temples in his palms.

Sometimes, through the vents that connected her bedroom to the living room, we would hear her sob and shout. "This is *my* house. It's *mine!*"

·4·

In June of 1989, my mother and father joined us for dinner with my in-laws from Oregon. My mother tried hard to practice the formalities of dinners and reunions, the greeting, the "Nice to see you," the kiss and hug at evening's end. But she sat silently throughout the meal, able to observe only that the corn tasted good.

In the living room, after dishes were cleared, she chose the chair farthest from the group, though we tried to pull her in. Soon, she disappeared for ten minutes to look at the roses. And then, for thirty more to talk to my parrot on the porch. "Look at the beautiful green leaves he has. Count them," I heard her say to some companion. But it wasn't me.

She made it through the evening, even drying a few pans, though she had no idea where they belonged or what they even were anymore. She knew only that rubbing them would make them shine, and she liked that.

I drove my parents home about 9:00 P.M. My father sat in the front with me. That was a mistake. As we talked—about my in-laws, my son's summer plans, my father's cataracts—I noticed in the rearview mirror that my mother's face was twisting in alarm. We tried to ask her simple questions, to include her, to make her our centerpiece. She only scrambled angry responses.

"You two can go to *hell!*" she finally said, crying so hard that she almost choked. I had never in my life heard my mother swear before. My father just shook his head.

When we entered their house, my mother ran to her room. Father told me not to go up. She had spells like this and it was best to let them pass, he said. She would forget everything by morning.

But I could not ignore her grief. She never had ignored mine when I had occupied the room that now was hers. I found her curled up in a corner of her closet, crying from the bottom of a canyon, holding a checkbook from a bank that had closed five years ago. I pushed her dresses far down the wooden bar and sat beside her. I rocked her in my arms and whispered that everything would be all right.

"He wants me out so he can have the house!" she cried. "I'm going to kill myself. I am."

"He doesn't want the house, Mother," I said, foolishly trying to reason with her. "He wants *you.*"

She did not understand. But finally she rose from the corner, from the closet, and perched herself on the edge of her bed. I sat beside her again, stroking her blond hair, so real amidst the blond veneer of the cheap furniture in her room. I helped her fold down the covers, hang up her blouse, undo the pins she had fastened on different parts of her underwear to hold it together. I draped her in the soft folds of a blue nightgown, and then curled up under her arm and rested with her. I wanted her to remember that I was her child. That I needed her.

"What's wrong?" I asked, not knowing why I even spoke.

"Everything," she said, turning away from me.

I left because there was nothing else I could think to do. Nothing at all.

I called early the next morning. My father was cheerful. "She's fine!" he assured me. "Doesn't even remember we had dinner with you!" I didn't know if his words were for me, or for him, or for her. But they softened the evening before.

I puzzled over my father's strength as I placed the phone in its cradle.

·5·

In 1991, the spring after my mother moved to Tanglewood, she nearly wrecked a bus.

She was still occasionally able to take short bus trips during the afternoons to ice cream stands, pretty sections of town, historic neighborhoods. Or so everyone thought. But she was about to make her final trip.

In the bus, I was told, she panicked. She wanted out and she fought her way to the front, scratching, kicking, beating arms and slapping faces. It took the strength of three professionals to restrain her, to hold her down until the bus pulled as rapidly as it could into the parking lot. She quivered all the way back, and well into the afternoon of her return.

Something in her dying and crazed brain had told her to run for her life. And she had had no choice but to obey.

·6·

When I arrive, my mother is standing by the nurse's station, angry. Nothing has happened, I am told. It's just not a good day for Annabelle. I give her my hand, but she refuses it. She rips strips of newspaper from section A.

Finally, she decides to move. She pinches my arm, hard, and pulls me down the hall. She turns toward the patio but completes the last few steps to the door almost on tiptoe, afraid of something I will never know. I reach to press the handlebar, breaking the seal. I step outside, but my mother has pulled away.

"Come with me, love," I motion.

She advances, stepping across the threshold to grab a handful of last fall's leaves. But when I fold her hand in mine to lead her down the patio sidewalk, she begins striking my arm, my shoulder, my chest with her fists. She slaps my face. I have never been struck before in my life.

She falls to her knees and creeps quickly back inside on her thin elbows. I feel the sting of my skin, the sting of my tears. I close the door and back up against the wall to brace myself, and wait to see what my mad mother will do next.

"Night!" she screams, her eyes wider than I have ever seen them in my life, an entire constellation of fear. "Gee night. Oh!" Her hands are visibly trembling, and so are mine. Bits of leaves seep from between her fingers and scatter onto the rug. She rises and stomps toward the living room and the nurse's station. There she furiously crushes the remaining leaves across the counter, spreads them, and tries to rub them into the veneer with her thumbs.

A nurse patiently waits until my mother turns in a new direction, then softly sweeps the leaves into a small pile and removes them from sight. "Do you need help?" she gently calls to me as we move away. "No," I say, too sharply, too proud to admit the truth that I'm afraid, physically afraid, of Annabelle Coyne.

Annabelle finds a favorite chair and sits. I sit beside her, and we make up. She rubs my leg and strokes my arm from shoulder to wrist. She twists the ring on my right hand, not even knowing that it's her own mother's wedding band, or her own husband's fractured diamond soldered on top. We close our eyes and rest.

·7·

I remember the night I knew I had no choice but to admit my mother.

My husband and I had started hiring a nursing service to stay with her at night so that we could sleep. She was confusing night and day and would often wander the house after midnight, sometimes turning on burners, sometimes finding a way to exit even when the doors were locked. Police would be called and bright lights from squad cars would beam across the dark streets of the neighborhood like Hollywood spots looking for a star. It was an all too familiar scene.

But this night, this horrible night, my mother pushed her nurse out of the house and down the cement stairs of the porch. When we found Annabelle, she was quaking in a chair crying about the men in the bushes who had raped her. The nurse, seriously bruised, shaken almost as badly as Annabelle herself, had phoned us from the next door neighbor's house shortly after two in the morning. Annabelle had locked her out.

The next day, I found Tanglewood.

·8·

Esther is sitting at the nurse's counter when I arrive. She calls me over. The unit, she explains, must comply with federal regulations and have all family of residents sign a release for use of restraints.

I can hardly breathe. How can I allow this? Seldom were people restrained at Tanglewood. But occasionally I would arrive to find a man with a soft blue "posey"—a curious name for a kind of partial straitjacket—sitting forlorn in a chair. Or a woman strapped gently in a G/C, screaming gibberish in a voice both too young and too high for her. I had watched these people before. I knew there was no other way. I had seen what the disease was doing to them.

But restraints were for other residents, not my mother. It wasn't time. It couldn't be happening already.

Esther lets me refuse, and closes the book that waits for my signature. "All right," she says. "We'll do without." But during the second hour of my visit, she joins my mother and me on our meaningless walk through the unit.

"Some days she goes out the patio door in the winter eight times in a row. She doesn't know what season it is, honey. Fire regulations prohibit us from locking the doors. The alarm sounds and we always fetch her right away, but in those seconds alone, on the ice, in the snow. If she falls . . ." As her sentence breaks, Esther puts her strong arm around my mother's waist to turn her.

Esther finds my hand and rolls it up softly in her other palm. "She bites now," Esther says, stroking my hand like a precious coin when she feels me tense. "She kicks and chews and bites when she's agitated. She'll hurt someone—or be hurt herself." I of course know that what Esther says is all too true.

And I know what Esther is really telling me. When my mother was first admitted, we were warned that Tanglewood could not handle the very violent—and violence is one of the curious roads the disease takes. Should my mother injure other residents, she will be asked to leave, a child suspended from school. Or, if she falls, the disease will accelerate at a frightening rate and she will be lost to me forever.

There is no clear rhythm to my heart or ethics any longer. There is just a sheet of paper on the counter and my mother at my side, clinging to my hand like the child I once was. One hand says yes. The other says no.

Esther catches my wrist. "We'll make it read the way you want," she says. She begins to write. "To be restrained for no more than 15–20 minutes with a soft posey and/or G/C. Then, release and redirect. Do not put back unless *severely* agitated."

I find the dark straight line that asks me to chain this free and wonderful creature smiling toothless beside me with such hope and trust.

And I sign.

Across the street from Tanglewood is an amusement park. Each day in the summer, thousands of people board Ferris wheels, roller coasters, and bumper cars that snap electricity into the air. They swim in the adjoining lake, they boat, they picnic. At the booths, they throw balls into hoops, at stuffed animals moving on a conveyor belt, at bottles with numbers on the sides.

The park advertises statues of monsters, every variety of hot dog America has imagined and manufactured, a pirate ship where young children can swing and slide and ring bells, a carnival of mirrors, a mechanical lion that you can have your picture taken with for just a few dollars, restaurants with blue pop, and gift shops where losers from the arcades can buy souvenirs to help weave their lies about good luck and great fortune after they return home.

When the wind blows just right in the afternoon, you can hear the screams of people going faster, falling more quickly, spinning more rapidly than human beings were ever meant to. The roar of the crowd reaches the patio of Tanglewood at just such times. If you visit Tanglewood at night and stand on the patio, you can see fireworks and laser lights dance in the sky.

Thousands of people looking for fun stream by Tanglewood each day in vans and four-wheel-drive vehicles filled with kids. They spend the entire day at the amusement park and eat three meals there. They walk to the parking lot loaded down with souvenirs and streaked with sunburn on shoulders and cheeks.

They have flown spaceships and driven monstrous whirligigs. They are happy now. They have laughed and screamed and been amazed. Children fall asleep in back

seats, exhausted, with licorice on their lips and cotton
candy in their hair.

Heads of life-size bears crunch windshields from the
passenger seats where they are being held by tired moms.

There has been so much to do. For every single minute
of the last twelve hours, there has been something to do.

A long line of cars spills slowly onto the street, lights
on, like a procession moving through the wrong time zone.

CHAPTER NINE

∾

Trivial Pursuit

there'll be a singsong after lunch
come on ladies
let's sing the monday song:
monday
fun day
CAROL MALYON, *Emma's Dead*

·1·

As I enter the home, I know it's Friday. Accordion music drifts out of the central dining hall. Happy Hour with Dave has begun.

Every Friday afternoon, Dave plays the accordion and people who can still dance without much help do. Today I hear "She'll Be Comin' Round the Mountain." Verse after verse, some familiar, some improvised, brings loud voices and stomping of feet. "We'll be havin' chicken and dump-lin's when she comes," "She'll be wearin' pink pa-ja-mas when she comes," "We will kill the old red roost-er when she comes," "She'll have to see her grand-pa when she comes."

Finally, the closing verse begins. "We'll be singin' Hal-le-lu-jah when she comes." The cooks are swinging their partners at the back of the room. Right in front of Dave, seven or eight residents, some from Tanglewood, are dancing in a large circle with the activity director and clapping their hands.

Six residents stay behind in Tanglewood during Happy Hour because they no longer know how to behave, how to have this kind of fun, or what a happy hour even is anymore.

Annabelle Coyne is one of them.

·2·

Kathleen returns to Tanglewood from Happy Hour with Dave shortly after 3:00 P.M. "My legs hurt," she says as she gets ready to sit next to me. "I've been dancing."

My mother has been sleeping through Happy Hour.

"How was the music?" I ask.

"I've heard better," she says with a small snort. "But he sang. It was funny. They gave us some popcorn."

Benny sits on the other side of Kathleen. "I like you!" he says to her.

"You've made my day!" she tells him, sincerely. "I didn't know everybody loved me the way they do."

"That show was pretty entertaining," she continues. "A kind of harmonica. What do you call those things that go out?" She moves her hands apart and then close together.

"An accordion," I say.

"That's right!" she sighs. "You're smart."

"I like you!" Benny smiles at Kathleen once more.

"You've made my day, as the hearing goes," she tells him. "Sometimes you need all the friends you can get."

Kathleen spots the TV. "They always are taking walks," she says, seeing several residents move in front of her. "I'd like to take a walk to Washington by way of *that*." She points to the TV. "Why isn't it on?"

"What's going on in Washington?" she asks me. "I'd like to hear it. I'm on the Board up there. There have been a lot of presidents lately, haven't there? Doesn't seem very comforting."

Gloria has entered the room. "Have you seen a tall handsome guy? That's my husband Bill." No one answers or responds. "Nobody knows him? Heavens to Murgatroyd!" she says in disbelief, hearing somewhere in her echo chamber of a mind the Snagglepuss imitations of her children, raised on Hanna-Barbera. "He's real handsome. I heard the man that played the violin. Beautiful. Just *lovely*." She presses her cane in front of her and exits stage left.

"What's she talking about? What violin?" Kathleen asks me.

"Probably means the accordion," I say.

"I studied voice in Rome for three years," Kathleen explains. "I made my debut in La Scala."

"What did you sing?" I ask, amazed by her disclosure.

"Can't remember," she says, trying to think. "'Ave Maria,' maybe."

She pauses, remembering no more about her youth, but looking for something to say.

"My son John will be sailing here in his boat. He'll rent a car and come right up. That's the way he is. My husband's gone. It's awful. Brilliant mind. Wonderful doctor. Operated on hearts."

Mr. Miller stops beside Kathleen and tips his baseball hat in her direction. "Seems like a pretty nice guy," she notices.

Kathleen receives a mail call. A paper, *The Exponent*, is delivered to her. It's not the Washington news she had hoped for, but it's news.

"Is that from your church?" I ask.

"I don't know," she tells me, beginning to scan the front page. "Oh, yeah, here's the Pope!" She recognizes the Pope's picture on the front. "I'm getting stupider and stupider. Can't even recognize the Pope. And he hasn't changed since the beginning of time!"

Kathleen rests for a while and stares at her paper. She hears a branch strike a window and looks outside. "Look at those trees," she points.

"Don't you like them?" I ask her.

"I like them, but I keep thinking about the way it will be when it's time to prune them. That will take five years, won't it?" She laughs and I join in.

"I *really* like you!!" shouts Benny, extremely excited now.

"Thank you, thank you," responds Kathleen. "It's amazing how long that sun is lasting. When will they bring some food? Usually we have a nice omelette on a very pretty tray."

"Soon," I tell her, watching my mother's eyes begin to open. Very, very soon.

·3·

Families and staff bring residents their children's old toys. They are piled high on the table that forms the centerpiece to the living area. There are colored beads that slide up and down wire columns, six-piece jigsaw puzzles, beach balls, plastic geometric forms that you shove triangles and squares and circles into. Most things donated to the unit are for children under five.

Residents wander by the table, attracted to the colors and the slick plastic feel of objects. But very few understand the principles and purposes of the toys. They rarely pick them up.

Squares and triangles are the same in Tanglewood. There are no fine distinctions. It really doesn't matter whether jigsaw pieces click together, for they form a world residents no longer occupy.

No toy, no puzzle, is simple enough for here.

·4·

"What is the capital of Australia?" asks a new volunteer who knows little about Tanglewood residents.

"I used to know that," Clora says.

"It starts with a C," the volunteer prods, like a game show host.

"*Clora!*" says Clora, excited. Clora is serious.

"No," the volunteer says. "Try again." But no matter how long she waits, she cannot tease the answer out.

She senses something is wrong and tries a simpler question. And then, a simpler still. Finally she closes the box and eyes the beach ball on the table. She picks it up and starts to bat it from woman to woman in the circle around her. They laugh, sometimes miss, but sometimes hit the ball in the air and surprise themselves.

Trivial Pursuit is not a game for residents of Tanglewood.

·5·

Tuesday at 11:00 A.M. I find the unit spinning with activity. Helen stands at a table paring apples and dicing ripe bananas into mouth-size cubes. Angie is holding a glass canister of Lorna Doones and helping Helen arrange the pieces of fruit on paper plates for distribution to residents.

The men are huddled in a corner playing with a rubber horse-shoe set. They remember fields of green grass and picnics and groups of huge young men strutting and squatting. Their cheeks redden and they begin to clear their throats loudly and spit on the linoleum. An aide stands ready and pushes a mop in the direction of the sound.

Three people are sitting at a card table playing hangman and tic-tac-toe, remembering from somewhere how pencils form stick figures and X's and O's.

My mother is asleep, her mouth wide open and her cheeks sunk so deeply that at first I do not recognize the contours of her face. On one side of her sits Isabelle. Two chairs away on the other side, Kathleen. There is room for me.

"We want cookies!" Kathleen says loudly.

The activity director hears her and walks to her side. "Kathleen, you know you're diabetic. But you can have the apples and the bananas."

"Well, I haven't shown any sugar in years," Kathleen grunts.

"Have the fruit, Kathleen. It's summer and nothing tastes better anyway."

Ruth sits next to Isabelle at the end of a row of rockers. She leans to one side and slowly thumbs through a magazine with twisted fingers. Her mission seems to have come to an end when her gaze rests on a page decorated with flamingos.

Ruth's son arrives. He stares at her lovingly. She doesn't seem to know him, but is interested in the bag he's brought along. "I'm your son, Mom," he tells her, reaching in a McDonald's bag and pulling out a strawberry milkshake. "Here. It's for you! Just for you." It's a treasure.

He has earned Ruth's trust once more. She takes the shake and begins to suck through the straw her son has placed at the side of her mouth. As she sucks, I see her beside a pool in a black bathing suit with pink flamingos, a cool drink lightly frosting her perfectly tapered fingers.

"What's going on here besides apples?" Kathleen laughs.

Gene strolls into the living area, sits down, and waits to be served a piece of fruit. Today he wears a pocket protector in his favorite plaid shirt. It reads, "Chlor-Trimeton. Allergy Tablets."

The ten-year-old boy who volunteers in the summer has been helping pour juice. He spots Gloria dabbing nail polish unevenly and sits at her table.

"I was a science teacher," she tells him. "And here I am doing my nails!" She pauses to let her brain catch up with the irony of her observation, waving ten messy pink flashes of color over her head. "And what do you want to do when you grow up?" she continues. The boy smiles, but shrugs his shoulders in response to a question that is too difficult for this particular morning in his young life.

Gloria seems glad for the chance to offer advice. "Do something *interesting*," she says, enunciating each syllable of the last word because she senses its importance. "Drawing? An actor? Well, keep the smile. And add to it."

The boy, dressed in a T-shirt with a horse's head on the front and its rear and tail on the back, seems to be growing inches in his seat as Gloria speaks to him. His shoulders no longer fold forward but press firmly against the back of his chair.

"You have so much going for you," she explains. "Your smile, your intelligence. You have beautiful eyes. And I see from your shirt that you know how to ride horses. You have *skills*. Why, I hope we meet again!"

The activity director has seen the boy sit and recognizes an opportunity. She brings over two boxes of Basic Picture Words, two-sided cards that have easy words on one surface and bright pictures of simple objects on the other. The director shows Gloria and the boy how to play.

"Do you want to play games?" Gloria asks him without conviction, perhaps a little afraid that this game will not be easy, will not turn out so well.

The boy takes the boxes and selects a few cards. He senses how to turn them. Not the word, but the picture he positions in front of Gloria's eyes.

"What's this?" he asks her, pointing to an oval object on the front.

"A lemon!" she says.

"Nope. Guess again."

"A pear!"

"Nope, not a pear!"

"A map!"

The boy knows that Gloria has lost her focus now and gives her the answer. "An egg, Gloria!" he says. "An egg!"

He holds a card with a carrot in front of her. She remembers and says the word. The boy claps. And then a nickel, which she calls a coin.

Isabelle is patting my mother's right hand. I am patting the other. We are trying to coax her into our world. "She's my gal," Isabelle says. "We are pals together."

"I love you, Mom," I hear Ruth's visitor say a little too loudly, unashamed of his affection. Ruth has left her hand half over her mouth after wiping the final beads of milkshake from her lips with the napkin her son has given her. I hear nothing, but I see the words her son has just spoken to her form silently on her own lips. He sees this too.

"I'm going on vacation." The son gulps emotion back down his throat. "When I get home I'm going to see you. OK, sweetie? OK, baby? I wish I could stay longer. I'll come as soon as I get home. OK? A deal?" He rises and plants a sloppy kiss on her cheek. The sound cracks across the room. He has become as careless with his love as a child.

Gloria's young friend is also about to leave. His mother, who works at Tanglewood, has come to take him home for lunch. "I'll always remember you," she says, blowing him a kiss. "There's a young man that wants to be a *teacher*, I'll tell people!"

Mr. Miller nearly knocks the boy over in his hurry down the hall.

"Where are you going so fast?" Angie asks Mr. Miller while she helps the child regain his balance. "Home!" Mr. Miller shouts, as if summoning a phantom cab that has just pulled into the lobby of Tanglewood.

"Home is where the heart is," Angie calls out to him, waving, blowing a kiss to the boy and then to Mr. Miller.

Angie feels sorry for Ruth now that her son has left. She carries Perky into the unit for just such reasons. Angie takes Ruth's finger and pushes it under the bird's green breast. He hops on immediately. The bird seems to like her but suddenly spots the cage of the other birds across the room and wants to join them.

He flies toward it, but his wings are clipped and he lands in my mother's lap. Perky climbs up her skirt, up her blouse, across her shoulder to the cushion that supports her head. He walks up the cushion and perches on the wooden back of my mother's chair. My mother is too sleepy to focus on the bird but seems to sense that something nice has just happened. Annabelle smiles and yawns.

Perky eyes the cage once more and this time flies and lands.

"He loves a cage," the director laughs. "It's a safe haven."

·6·

Wednesday's activities:

9:00 A.M. Current Events
10:00 A.M. Rhythm Band and Exercise
11:00 A.M. Crafts in the Activity Room
2:00 P.M. Bus Ride
4:00 P.M. Stretching Activity
6:00 P.M. News Report
7:00 P.M. Game Shows
9:00 P.M. SWEET DREAMS

The bus ride is an especially popular treat. Because my mother is no longer invited, I sometimes feel like the parent of a youngster who is not allowed to go on a field trip, but I understand. When I visit during the bus ride, the unit is quiet and my mother is usually calm. It's a good time for a visit.

I have become Annabelle's only field trip.

Today Gloria has stayed behind too, stayed behind from the visit to the Thompkins Family Farm and the chance to pet dairy cows, refused to climb aboard. This is not normal. Gloria usually is eager to go anywhere at any time with anyone. But there she is sitting on a chair she's placed half in the hall, half in her room, waiting for Bill. Someone has told her he's gone golfing and will return soon.

Gloria will give up even the highlight of the week for a glimpse of Bill with his nine iron dangling over his shoulder.

·7·

There is a craft room in Tanglewood. In one corner is a commercial popcorn popper for Happy Hour. Larger toys also fill this room: a four-foot basketball stand, a stationary bike (which not a single person, in my experience, has ever used). And on tables are scraps of fabric, upholstery, donated paper yellowed by the sun, crayons and paints and glue, cotton and yarn and styrofoam cups.

Few residents can do crafts any longer. They don't understand how to follow sequences. At best, the room becomes an assembly line at 11:00 A.M. on Wednesdays. One person pastes, another tries to cut, someone else with agile hands ties knots. The tasks are simple, yet still impossible for many.

At the annual Christmas crafts show at The Woods in late November, Tanglewood items sell for less than items made by people who live in other wings of the complex. They are simple and not very beautiful.

Small lies are told to families about what Gene or Annabelle or Ruth made. We choose to believe them. We choose, just for an afternoon, to remember the former productivity of our relatives. We close our eyes and see our parents behind the wheels of automobiles and forklifts and trucks, snapping cards in a winning hand of bridge, hammering storm windows into place with heavy mallets, dusting cornmeal on counters.

Most items are made from cut-up magazines. Stationery with colorful squares pasted on the front (five packs for a dollar). Laminated bookmarks with ragged pictures of fruit or vegetables on one side. There are chalk drawings more primitive than a kindergartner's. Pictures of sheep on small pieces of art paper, made fragile by golden popcorn fleece glued to their bodies.

I buy these things foolishly, hungrily, with murderous greed.

I want my mother back.

·8·

For many years, I helped my mother with her Christmas cards. The year before she entered Tanglewood, I took her shopping for the cards and sat with her at her kitchen table as she looked up addresses and tried to remember who the people were behind the names of streets and numbers.

The first year after my mother was admitted, I bought the cards and printed address labels on my computer. My mother stuck the labels to the envelopes and signed her name. That year, too, I took her picture with my camera and she stuffed the cards with reprints.

The second year of my mother's residence, she could no longer sign her name, no longer read. I had a stamp made with the words "Annabelle Coyne" on it. She would hold the stamp and press it into the ink pad, then onto the thick paper of the card. Sometimes the name was upside down. She never noticed. I purchased self-adhesive return address labels for the envelopes. She had trouble deciding where to put the postage stamp, where the return label.

By her third year at Tanglewood, my mother had forgotten what cards and envelopes were for, had forgotten her own name. I tried to get her to at least lick the stamps, but I could do this only by holding her mouth open and pressing the American flag to her tongue.

My patriotism, my loyalty to the cause of wanting a normal Christmas and a normal mother, made her gag. My mother would not tongue a lie. She never had in her life.

After that, I gave up Christmas forever.

·9·

Something in the memories of old people keeps bingo alive long after other games have vanished from their heads. In Tanglewood, only a few residents can play bingo without help. Even the large, simpler boards are confusing. But aides place themselves strategically around the table and tell players when their numbers have been called. They shout "I-24!" and "G-6!" into deaf ears, waving huge cards with letters and numbers in the air. Sometimes they place chips made from milk container tops between arthritic fingers and help residents cover winning squares.

The shout of "BINGO!" electrifies the group. Even the disappointed losers come alive. To win bingo is something that matters. But just to play bingo is enough. It is a measure of mental superiority and identifies the leaders in the unit.

My mother hasn't played bingo for years.

"Thank you for playing, ladies," an aide will say, meaning it. "That was a super game." She'll clap for them.

When it's over, winners and losers receive vanilla wafers distributed from a large fish bowl. Next, a piece of soft candy wrapped in colored paper. Some women fill their pockets with these things. They hoard them. It's all the treasure that they have in the world.

In Tanglewood, former ideas of ownership vanish. Residents wander into rooms not their own, look in drawers of strangers, take whatever sparkles, trace the outlines of faces on other residents' photographs, wear shoes belonging to someone else. Knowing this, staff advise families to strip their mothers and fathers, their sisters and brothers, their sons and daughters, of engagement rings and wedding bands, of watches and jewelry.

Candy becomes sweeter than it ever was before.

CHAPTER TEN

❧

Sunday

*She was ready for church. She took Paul every Sunday
because what he couldn't get out of the sermon he
managed to get out of the hymns. According to Lois
he could sing a hymn all the way through when a
congregation was there to jump-start him.*

BEVERLY COYLE, *In Troubled Waters*

·1·

I arrive in mid-afternoon one Sunday early in the summer. It's
3:30 P.M. But the church service is still going on. I hear the
final crescendo of "How Great Thou Art." A woman in rose
eyelet, dressed and shaped like a spring tulip, is standing by the
piano waving her arms, one hand grasping the *Bible Song and
Promise Book*. Beside her is a younger version of herself, a bud,
perhaps a daughter, also dressed in bright rose. The daughter is
playing the violin, and the notes swell with the voice of the older
woman.

The woman asks for applause for the violin player. Some people in the unit eagerly do as they're told. Isabelle, the apricot princess today, is still dressed at 3:30 P.M. in her soft orange bathrobe, ruffled at the collar and sleeve in white. She claps loudly.

"And let's not forget Jesus!" the woman in rose reminds them. "Let's give him a hand too." Fewer people respond, beginning to rub their eyes or wander down halls. They remember the shrill violin of just moments before. And some lines from the songs chosen by the woman still cling to the few healthy neurons floating in their brains. The lines have been encoded in their heads from all those church services, all those noontime radio hymns women ironed to in the '50s and the '60s.

But Jesus fled Tanglewood a long time ago.

·2·

"How did you like church today?" I ask Isabelle as the woman in rose folds her music stand, gathers her belongings, and once more praises her assistant on the violin.

"I didn't go," she tells me. "I didn't get up in time. I was late this morning. I was rushing around doing the dishes and Pete . . ." Her sentence stops.

"Did you go?" Isabelle asks Kathleen, seated beside her.

"Oh, yes!" Kathleen responds. "It was so nice and peaceful. I especially liked seeing the children and hearing the children's sermon." She sits and rocks, seeing something in a northern suburb of her past, not here.

Gloria spots me and somehow thinks I'm part of the church group today. "What a nice surprise to see you and your other friends!" she shouts across the room. "This is my first visit. I just love it! I'll be here every day!"

We all will, I think. Sooner or later, we all will.

·3·

Anna Golz, my mother's mother, belonged to the German-speaking congregation of Zion Lutheran Church in Akron from the time of her arrival in the United States. Around 1904, Pastor Yount started the missionary congregation known as Concordia Evangelical Lutheran Church—an English-speaking church. Many of the Golzes, including Anna and her family, transferred their membership to Concordia.

In 1905, when the first church was built, it actually adjoined the backyard of the Haberkost home. It remained there until 1923 when a new church was erected down the street. One of Annabelle's uncles, Leo Golz, was the general contractor for that structure. The husband of Anna's sister Ida, Albert Koehn, did all the roofing and the sheetmetal work.

Annabelle was baptized on October 2, 1910, baptized, literally, in her own backyard. She was married on July 25, 1936, in the church her uncle helped to build, the church where I would marry thirty-three years later.

To the best of my knowledge, Annabelle never missed a Sunday. She was dutiful to the church. My father, a lapsed Catholic, started accompanying her to Concordia after he retired.

My mother never talked about God with me. But as a young girl I remember the times she refused communion, punishing herself, or others, in ways I could not then comprehend.

Church, then brunch, became the rituals my mother and father practiced longest. I remember my father telling me why they stopped attending services. My mother would sing too loudly at the wrong times and eye people next to her with suspicion and hostility.

So brunch became the last ritual they were faithful to in the final days—eggs and white toast and fried potatoes sizzling on the grill.

·4·

Sunday brunch is about to be served and Millie is leafing through magazines again. Magazines are her obsession. This time she thumbs through *St. Anthony Messenger*. On a full page she spots an ad for a holy porcelain figurine. "Ave Maria!" she reads, placing a paper napkin on her head and laughing through broken teeth.

Maggy is on duty, pumping hard to finish Millie's blood pressure before plates are set on the table. "OK," Maggy shouts, doing two things at once, "who will pray for us before we eat?"

Kathleen, who always says the prayer before meals, volunteers as if for the first time.

In a single breath, the words spill from her mouth into the room. "Bless us, O Lord, and these thy gifts which we are about to receive, through thy bounty, from Christ our Lord, Amen!"

She breathes hard and quickly for a moment and then looks at her empty cup. "Hey!" she continues. "I'd like to have my coffee now, if you don't mind!"

·5·

"She's my baby doll," Isabelle tells me one Sunday in July, patting my mother's hand. Isabelle is dressed as the apricot princess again today. "She's not only from my church, you know. She would help me with all my household chores."

Isabelle is the one woman in the unit that my mother will let fuss over her. In the mornings when Annabelle sometimes comes to breakfast in her nightgown and a staff member tries to head her back toward her room to change, Isabelle defends my mother's rights. "Don't hurt my baby doll!" she yells, sometimes poking and hitting an attendant who gently ignores her.

"Do you want to stay or leave?" she asks my mother. "She's in my section," she tells me. "Doesn't her hair lay down nicely today? Sometimes we have trouble with it. She's so pretty. We work together sometimes, don't we?" She runs her fingers through my mother's hair and Annabelle closes her eyes and dreams.

"Did you eat?" she persists, looking directly into my mother's eyes. "Or don't you remember? Did you have lunch or breakfast today? Count 'em up: breakfast, lunch, and dinner! We need them all, you know. We need all three!"

"She has been with us a long time," Isabelle continues, apparently sure that she has hired my mother to work for her in her life before Tanglewood. "We tell each other stories."

Mr. Miller is sitting with Esther behind the nurse's station. "When's this wedding supposed to start?" he leans over to ask Esther.

Esther, smiling and amused, says that there's no wedding today in Tanglewood that she knows about. That is, unless Mr. Miller has some plans of his own.

"Well, what the hell's this all about then?" he asks, annoyed, wondering why nurses are wheeling patients from other units into the living area of Tanglewood. Two, three, then five and more are whisked into the unit and abandoned.

"It's church," Esther explains. "It's 2:30 P.M. Sunday and we always have church, Mr. Miller."

A minister with camel hair and camel sportcoat flings open the doors of Tanglewood, and enters. Behind him is a small caravan of older women and teens, carrying Bibles, music stands, and brown and black cases filled with sacred objects from another world. One teen with stacks of red curls immediately makes her way toward the piano, softly stroking the hair of residents as she winds through chairs. The older women from the church greet members of their new congregation.

A woman dressed in glossy cobalt passes out slender hymnals printed just for services at the home. My mother and Isabelle, sitting along the wall far from the improvised church, are coaxed to join, but refuse. "You are her daughter, aren't you?" the woman from church asks me. "You have the same unusual blue eyes. I've never seen such eyes."

She leans toward me like an optician. I take a hymnal and thank her, lowering my head to the songs.

" 'In the Garden,' " the woman in cobalt proclaims. "That was surely your favorite song once, remember?" she speaks to the group, for the group.

The piano begins and the woman makes sure those who can

turn pages have found page five. Most residents just stare at the words that begin the song, the voices of the people from other units and from the church dominating the sing. But when the refrain begins, scratches of old sound, like 78 records, enter in. "And He walks with me, and He talks with me, And He tells me I am His own, And the joy we share as we tar-ry there, None oth-er has ev-er known!"

"Second verse!" the leader yells out. But second verses are deep mysteries in Tanglewood, and feet tap nervously until the refrain begins and residents know they're home. A few can still see the windows of their own churches and smell the summers that once floated through them into their pews.

The leader opens her Bible to Luke and finds the story of the criminal on the cross. "'And he said unto Jesus, Lord, remember me when thou comest into thy kingdom.'" She helps people turn to page six. "Now sing out 'Jesus, Remember Me'!" she shouts, naming the next song.

My mother and Isabelle are busy loving each other. Isabelle rubs her hand sweetly and my mother smiles. "We go by smiles here," she explains. "She's all right if you see a smile." Isabelle pauses briefly and then turns her attention once more to my mother. "Will you walk with me and see if you like it?" she asks Annabelle. But my mother does not want to walk to church this afternoon. Not even with Isabelle.

"Good! Very good!" the leader encourages her congregation at the end of the second hymn. She approaches Benny and asks him why he's not singing today. "We need all the basses we can get around here!" she explains. Benny thinks she's flirting with him and tries to pinch her breast.

"'What a Friend We Have in Jesus'!" The third hymn of the service is selected. Behind the nurse's station Mr. Miller still sits, enjoying his power. He has only a vague sense of what is going on. "Death must be OK," he tells Esther, "because nobody has ever come back from it!" It's one of his favorite lines. He says it over and over. It's a joke he's shared with men over morning coffee and toast a hundred times. His laugh echoes from every corner of the room until the music begins again.

"Sing it out!" the leader urges. Most lines are mumbled, but "Take it to the Lord in prayer" and "Ev-ery-thing to God in prayer" drown out even the piano. I wonder how many of the men and women in Tanglewood still are able to pray, or remember what that old habit is about. I wonder what God thinks when their scrambled messages reach heaven.

"'The Old Rugged Cross'! You probably know the words by memory," the woman in cobalt announces. Some people nod before their indecipherable groans begin like the chants of monks and they wait for the chorus.

My mother has risen and is walking to the edge of the group. The minister begins his sermon. He tells us that he had had one sermon prepared but Sunday School and the woods outside the Tanglewood windows have put him in mind of something else. "When I was a boy," he begins, "I loved the woods. They were woods like those." He points out the window. "I would swing on a grapevine tied to an old tire. Do you remember doing that?"

Some residents nod. Others pick scabs or drift off to sleep.

"But one day I found myself lost in those woods. Lost. I forgot where I was. We have to come to a point when we realize we're lost. That's the way it was in my Christian life too. The Bible says we're lost without Jesus. The Spirit spoke to me. Then I got scared. I never wanted to be lost like that again."

My mother has begun pushing a woman in a wheelchair out of the circle, but the woman doesn't seem to care. I distract Annabelle and return the chair to its position.

"It's in the Second Letter of Paul to the Corinthians, Chapter 4. We have the power from God. 'Hard-pressed on every side, we are never hemmed in; bewildered, we are never at our wits' end; hunted, we are never abandoned to our fate; struck down, we are not left to die.'"

He rests a minute. "What is our peace?" he asks the group. "Can you tell me?"

Mrs. Blackburn waves her hand and shouts, "Why, the resurrection, of course!"

"The resurrection! Yes, the resurrection!" he says, calling her words into the room like the numbers on a bingo card.

"We drove over here today," the minister continues. "We could have had a fatal accident on the way. We don't know if we have even one more hour of life. Not one more hour. We can't be sure."

The minister backs up and the woman in cobalt begins her testimony. "I think standing here that I'll be where you are someday. We are all the Lord's. He knows if you're angry, or if you're in pain. God doesn't take the pain away sometimes, but gives us grace to sustain it. Hold onto the thought that God is up there waiting for you. God will take care of you. Jesus will remember you!"

People are growing restless, so the piano begins again and the leader takes requests. "I Love to Tell the Story" and then "O God, Our Help in Ages Past" as an encore.

My mother has also become restless, wandering into her room. She looks at a picture of the Virgin Mary resting in a transparent frame on her dresser. The virgin is draped in black and modestly pulls a fold of fabric over one cheek. I have never seen this picture in her room before. The virgin decorates a Catholic interment announcement for someone my mother does not know, an announcement that has wandered into my mother's room in the middle of the night. Annabelle stares at it hard. "Caniglia and Sons Funeral Home," I read on the back as my mother examines the picture on the front.

Next my mother spots her table lamp, a tall bronze thing whose base twists upward like a giant spiral candle, topped by a white cylindrical shade. It is unplugged, as if it has been waiting for her. She slides it down the dresser top and into her arms. She holds it with both hands at a forty-five degree angle, like a flagpole, a candle snuffer, an incense post. She has become an altar boy, an acolyte, and wanders slowly and ceremoniously down the hall toward the church service.

It is a holy moment. The last phrase about "our e-ter-nal home" floats in the air. Some people have stopped to stare at my mother. Some of the staff giggle. A few residents grow disgusted and angry. The church people are confused.

Isabelle spots Annabelle and smiles from one deaf ear to the other. She guides my mother to the center of the room, placing her directly under the sun roof carved into the cathedral ceiling, bronze chandeliers with electric candle bulbs on either side. A beam beats onto the top of her blond hair, setting it on fire.

"Well . . . well, hello!" another woman from the church awkwardly greets my mother. She tries to touch her, but my mother's hands are occupied with the lamp and her body is buried behind it. The woman's hands flutter uncomfortably around my mother's body and head and then return to her side. "God bless you. God bless you, dear lady."

Annabelle receives her blessing and turns away. She shuffles like an ancient priest down the hall, with the base of the lamp pressed firmly into her stomach, the light extinguished forever.

CHAPTER ELEVEN

Transformations

"I'm going to get Lisa's present out of the refrigerator," says my grandmother.
The refrigerator?
NANCY WHITELAW, A *Beautiful Pearl*

·1·

My mother winds her way into another resident's room. I'm on her arm. A television is blaring from the dresser where it sits. But no one is in the room. On an afternoon talk show Maury Povich is interviewing fat women who have lost weight.

"I used to weigh three hundred pounds," says a pencil-thin woman who looks like a New York model.

Maury holds up the "before" picture of the woman for the camera to see.

"Can you believe these two people are the same?" he asks, inanely. "It's a miracle. A miracle!"

·2·

Before my mother came to live at Tanglewood, she lost or ruined several hearing aids. She knew to take the hearing aids out of her ears at night, but she had forgotten how to store them. Many mornings we would find them swimming in the Efferdent water of her denture case. Rust would form, corroding batteries and ruining the delicate systems inside.

Even after she came to Tanglewood, it became impossible to help her understand. The hearing aids would show up in glasses of milk, other people's jewelry boxes, planters of flowers, the fish tank.

Eventually insurance companies dropped her.

Her disease progressed more rapidly because the world now began to roll out like a silent film. Worse. Even the piano that provided a melody line in the background of the films could not reach her profoundly deaf ears.

Next, her teeth became a mystery to her. She began to refuse them, to take them out when nurses weren't looking. We found them buried in snowdrifts, sitting on windowsills, resting on racks inside the stove in the Tanglewood kitchen.

They were not a part of her, really. And she knew it. She tried to figure out what they were again and again until one day they grew too puzzling and they disappeared altogether.

She got rid of the problem, and we'll never know how she did it.

Two years after she came to live at Tanglewood, my mother had only four original molars to grind her food with, and was stone deaf.

·3·

The alarm rings in Tanglewood for two reasons. First, when a resident goes outside or into the nursing wing through one of the three sets of doors. Second, when a resident forgets how to flush a toilet and pulls down the help cord instead of the silver handle on the porcelain bowl.

·4·

Louie, the woman in yellow, my mother's roommate, wants to be in television. What she sees on the television screen in the corner of the room is more real to her now than anything that happens in the unit where she lives. Louie would stand in front of the TV twelve hours a day if it were on, with her stuffed animals in her arms. People have to tell her to sit down.

Even when she sits she draws her chair up as close to the screen as she can without inciting someone's anger, and snuggles up. She can't resist touching the stand or maybe, if she gets close enough, a button or a knob.

It's after two and *Captain Planet* is on. A horrible oil spill has occurred and mutant purple globs of goo have begun to form and seep into the city where the Planeteers live. The purple globs, great gelatinous dinosaurs, find their way into any area with dirt or garbage. They roll into cars and suck out ashtrays with their malformed snouts. They raid garbage cans and dream of landfills.

This is a job for Captain Planet. The Planeteers summon him by reciting magic words as they aim their rings into the air. "Earth, fire, water, wind, heart!" they scream. The combination of forces makes Captain Planet visible, for he is made of all these things.

"Soon there will be nothing left but a planet of living garbage," Captain Planet mourns.

A commercial interrupts. This is Louie's favorite part. No one wants to watch during the commercial, except Louie, so she stands steady, owning the television. She grabs for the Cocoa Pebbles and holds her arms out when she sees a beach ball flying through the air. She would like to climb in. She prefers color to black and white.

Ronald McDonald pulls a lampshade over his head and it lights up. The picture blackens, Louie is ordered to sit down, and Captain Planet returns to the screen.

Captain Planet uses the force of all the elements, and heart, of course, to destroy the purple blobs and gobs. They cannot resist his power now. He saves the Planeteers as purple tentacles grab their cruiser. The purple worms wind helplessly into a clear cylinder that changes into a propeller as the hero spins it madly in the air.

I twist my ring and wish and wish for Captain Planet.

Louie knows her turn has once again come. The cartoon has ended. She stands inches from the screen and presses her palms directly on it, static snapping through the room. Eggos are advertised. They pop from a toaster and fill the picture. A boy pours streams of maple syrup over them. The syrup spills into the squares of the waffle, overflowing.

Louie opens her mouth and licks every inch of the screen, even after the syrup is gone and replaced by previews for the next cartoon.

·5·

It's Family Night. The staff has assembled and is telling family visitors how residents have spent their summer vacations. We hear about bowling and bingo, about the wedding shower and fashion show, about bus rides and conversations. On the wall behind the activity director is a huge circle of green cardboard—the Tanglewood family tree. On it are five-by-seven photos of residents. Beside Angie is a table of wonderful sweets, cookies and cakes and orange punch and truffles in every flavor dripping with ribbons of sweet icing.

After explanations and introductions, we all are invited to do the Alleycat, the favorite dance at Tanglewood. The music begins and Angie sways to the right, sways to the left, steps forward, steps backward. The residents begin to imitate her, and so do we. Before long, Faye finds the director's waist and holds on tight and then a few others link behind her. Arms and hips are swaying in every corner of the unit and no one is old.

The videotape of the wedding is inserted after visitors and residents have returned from the table of sweets. No one in the unit remembers the occasion, but a few, the very best bingo players, recognize themselves and feel famous.

Most are only confused by the playback. Reality was unknowable the first time, and the playback is impossible to understand.

Kathleen sits and talks with the activity director, her back turned to the screen as she meets the director's eyes. Kathleen does not see herself on the tape, but there she is in celluloid, rocking, being interviewed by Angie. She hears Angie's questions from several days before. "What was the color of your dress at your own wedding?" "The color of your bridesmaids' dresses?" "Where were you married?"

It doesn't seem peculiar to Kathleen that the lips of the Angie she now faces are not moving. She hears the questions float into the room and answers them the same way she had when they were first posed to her, creating a duet with the soundtrack behind her: "white, don't remember, Woodlawn Avenue." Angie has become a ventriloquist, that's all.

Mrs. Blackburn is urged by several aides to look at the screen when her image appears. She seems unmoved, uninterested. "That's you!" they tell her. "No it's not," she responds as she turns and finally spots the screen. "That's not me. I don't have that on today."

I smile in her direction and she talks to me. "They built ten houses around the corner from our confectioner's shop in New York City. Just for the movies. That was when movies were just starting out. They would make movies and then every night they wanted maple ice cream. Maple ice cream made me popular, and rich." Mrs. Blackburn rocks slowly and glances back up at the screen. She is still there on tape, dressed in the argyle sweater that has confused her. She finally seems to understand.

"There!" she cries, tapping my shoulder and pointing to the

screen with her slender and perfect finger. "I was so popular, with the boys too, that one night they put me in their movie. See, there I am! The very, *very* pretty one."

·6·

Gloria has decided to become the choir director for the afternoon. She sits at a table sorting through music, eventually landing upon a songbook titled *Happy Days Are Here Again*. She has made her decision and heads toward the piano with this single treasure under her arms. Other volumes of songs will remain closed today.

Standing beside the piano, Gloria opens the book to the middle and begins to hum and direct. Her cane swings in front of her triangular body like the steel pointer on a metronome. It is pitchless Gregorian chant she sings. Occasionally a piercing note flies unexpectedly through her lips and drills itself into a healthy ear.

She grows impatient. No one will join her group in spite of her pleas between songs. "Come forward! Don't be shy! Sing with me!" No recruits today. Nonetheless, the third song, as unrecognizable and unmelodious as the first, is about to begin under the baton of Gloria the conductor.

My mother does not notice Gloria, does not hear her, but she does find the piano interesting at this very moment for some reason and travels toward it, full steam. She stops in front of it, Gloria watching her with suspicion but still humming relentlessly.

Annabelle lowers her head and lifts her hand in the air. Her fingers slam onto the black keys. They never touch the white keys but move from black to black all the way to the top, all the way to a badly out of tune note that resembles the shrill and dissonant squawks that now and then escape through Gloria's mouth. The white keys may as well not be there.

Gloria accepts Annabelle as her accompanist. Their eyes never meet, but it is a perfect duet. It is New Music they make, all avant-garde, where noise and silence become sound, where chance plays a part, where chromatic scales anoint the air.

·7·

Within arm's reach over the patio fence is a clump of tall black-eyed Susans. I pluck a blossom and give it to my mother. She shows no interest in it today. I stuff it in a buttonhole of my blouse.

After we return to the unit, I see Gert. Gert, as usual, is making an irritating buzzing sound through her vibrating lips.

"Hi, Gert!" I say.

She buzzes more rapidly, like a bee, sending spit across the room.

"Here," I say, loosening the orange and black flower from my clothes. "Isn't this pretty?"

Gert takes the flower by the stalk, blinks her eyes in wonder, and in one gulp bites the head off and chews.

·8·

Faye is walking happily down the hall arm in arm with Betty Jane. She stops to greet me.

"So, what's new, Faye?" I ask her.

"Well," she says, out of breath, "have you met Grandma?"

"No," I tell her.

She puts her arm around Betty Jane's shoulder and introduces Grandma to me.

"Grandma and I were just in a room talking," she goes on. "We hardly get a chance to do that anymore."

Betty Jane—Grandma in Faye's eyes—smiles in agreement. "This is the first time I've been here," Betty Jane, a three-year resident, tells me. "And it sure is nice."

Faye is a girl again, happy learning secrets from her grandma, happy feeling young beside this ancient woman she thinks is eight times her age.

·9·

Annabelle is confused today, confused by every item in her small world. She is restless. I see her heart beating in the broad veins of her neck.

She spots Isabelle's cane across the room and joins her. My mother removes Isabelle's shoe and tries to attach it to the hook of the cane. She tries to thread cane into the toe, the heel. It won't stay.

Isabelle doesn't mind. She pampers my mother. "Want me to try it?"

My mother has not looked up, but her eyes are swollen with alarm.

"I'll bet you a cookie you can do it! That's nice!" Isabelle praises her. "Thank you!" The shoe finally dangles precariously from the wooden cane. "Atta boy!" Isabelle smiles.

My mother returns the shoe to Isabelle and now tries to force the tip of the cane under the tongue of her own shoe.

"You can use that if you want to," Isabelle tells Annabelle. Annabelle stands and takes the cane with her, holding it with both hands like a tap dancer would. She shuffle-ball-changes her way across the room.

My mother looks for a place to sit. She roams over toward the magazine table. On each side of it is a small row of pink vinyl armchairs that are very popular in the unit. Several are unoccupied. Along with three magazines, a wrought iron lamp approximately three feet high rests on the surface of the table.

Annabelle looks at the arrangement, puzzled. Then she turns and begins backing up. She has figured the world out as best she can today. She very deliberately sits on the table, nearly upsetting the powerful lamp.

"Hey, you can't do that! What are you doing?" some of the other residents complain. Annabelle does not hear them. They jab her rear, trying to push her off, but she clenches the sides with her strong arms and resists. The cane falls noisily to the floor.

The dance is over. But Annabelle stays put.

·10·

When I arrive, Annabelle is roaming the unit dressed in her purple sweat suit and carrying an enormous vinyl cushion with bright flowers that belongs in the wicker chair. She clearly has some plan, some purpose in mind. She lets me kiss her but refuses to release her colorful package. She seems content holding it, happy almost, and skates down the hall clutching it close to her braless chest.

Finally, my mother sees a vacant chair in the living room and carefully backs into it. She places the pillow on her lap and taps it several times into place. It might have been a great, flowered Ouija board. The seats to her right and to her left are already occupied, so I crouch in front of her and place my arms on the flowered surface.

Slowly, hands begin to crawl onto the cushion and it comes alive. Louie, seated to my mother's right, sees my arms and moves her hand toward my watch, the magical planchette for the game we are about to play. She twists the band, feels the small chain, and rubs the glass. "Pretty," she smiles. "That's pretty." Ruth, on the other side of my mother, sporting long red nails that match the red frames of her glasses, races her nearly transparent fingers to my other hand and begins to trace my bones.

My mother takes her hands and runs them up and down my arms several times, from shoulder to fingertip, bending her back to reach me. She does this again and again, bumping over the hands of Louie and Ruth with each trip. She stops and lifts the little finger of my right hand, twisted curiously out of shape exactly as hers is, twisted from birth by a common gene. The finger suddenly seems more familiar to her than my face and she moves her eyes closer to study it.

This is an ancient game we play.

When my mother at last sweeps the cushion clear, she senses that its purpose has been served. She slides it vertically between two chairs and abandons it.

Now, as she moves rapidly across the room, going nowhere, it is only my hand she holds tightly in her own.

CHAPTER TWELVE

❧

Sundowning

*This was a busy time of day for the hot line people.
In the late afternoon all caregivers had a higher rate
of incidents. For one thing there was "sundowner's
syndrome" in the late afternoon. Everything about
everyone's situation seemed worse as darkness fell.
Everyone took turns not knowing where they were.*
BEVERLY COYLE, In Troubled Waters

·1·

Last winter, a woman from a famous clinic came to study
the behavior of Tanglewood residents between 4:30 P.M.
and 8:00 P.M. Sundowning occurs during these hours, and
the woman was gathering urine samples to see if any medical
changes could be recorded that would explain the strange things
that begin with the downswing of the clock in late afternoon.
Some theorists think that sundowning might be a biochemical
response to the fading of daylight.

The Criers begin to cry harder as the sun goes down. Screamers scream more loudly. Repeaters howl their questions and demands even more rapidly into the air. The Restless, like my mother, quiver in madness and move on high. Evening Crazies stagger everywhere.

The woman studied residents for several months, found nothing very significant, and left. She did make one recommendation, though. Now Tanglewood has new fluorescent lights in all the hallways.

The nurses haven't noticed any difference.

·2·

When my mother lived with us during my father's illness, I prayed the sun would never set. But it always did.

Around five o'clock, her eyes would glaze strangely, and she would head toward the south windows in our kitchen to find the garage. There she spotted my father's car. She would race out the back door and down the drive, climb in the driver's seat, and travel home without starting the engine. She hadn't driven for five years, but she had taken up driving again now that my father was ill.

At first I let her drive in the garage. But each day it would be harder to pry her from the seat at the end of her trip and unfasten her arms from their embrace of the wheel. Minutes of play turned into excruciating hours of worry. On the Friday of the second week of her long trip home, it took four people to remove my mother, screaming, from the red leather seat of her '88 Oldsmobile.

After that, I began locking the kitchen door. But she took the screens out from the window next to it, shot herself through, and bolted toward her red ticket home.

Next, I locked the car, and found her crying tears onto the windshield, helplessly looking in, her arms moving rhythmically from side to side, like wiper blades.

One day, in twilight, I gave up. I knew I would soon have to sell my father's car. For now, I parked it down the street, out of view.

My mother spent late afternoons staring from the kitchen window through empty eyes into the empty shell of the garage where her chariot had once been. Perhaps it would return for her in a blaze, with my father at the wheel once more, in his red driver's hat and paisley ascot, hair slicked back with Vitalis, Big Band music playing in quadraphonic, hailing her with a hey and a ho and a "Hey, Annabelle!"

In twilight, my mother cannot win. Neither can I.

· 3 ·

It is 7:00 P.M. when I arrive. My mother is restrained in a G/C with a soft posey. At sundown, poseys come out, the evening primrose of Tanglewood. She is pulling herself forward with all her weight and strength, and then flying back like a rubber band from the elastic strips that bind her. I untie the knot at the back and pull her up.

She has the energy and obstinacy of a five-year-old tonight. She refuses her shoes, refuses everything. She tightens her lips when the nurse brings her medications, and spits out what little trickles through.

She races down the halls, charging into anyone in her way. She carelessly threads her body through tables and chairs without noticing walkers, people out for a stroll, carts.

She is busy beyond belief. She locates a captain's chair and pushes it toward the main entrance. There she pauses for just a moment to feel the molding on the steel doors and to clump the lace curtains into ponytails. She pushes the chair back into the unit, a powerful caboose that's lost its engine.

She tours the patio, shoeless, seven or eight times. She drops to her knees and crawls up the cement walkway to the door of the unit. She stands and enters.

She steals three canes and two walkers, women yelling at her and saying they will beat her up. Everything is returned, in time.

Several women are watching *Jeopardy*, the unit's favorite night-time TV show, the show that burned its way into their living

IN A TANGLED WOOD

rooms for years and years before someone sold their houses and moved them to Tanglewood. The host is introducing guests from New York and Minnesota and California for the evening's round. "The best and the brightest," he calls them. They proceed to choose categories in Science and Russian Literature and Politics, and to recall names like Elliot Richardson with ease.

My mother prowls outside rooms where the Sweet Dreams shift is changing beds. She snatches dirty linen and mattress covers that have been tossed in doorways for later disposal. Aides scratch their heads in wonder when they exit, until they see Annabelle streaking away from them, like a sprite, with bundles under her arms.

In her room, she takes stuffed animals and dolls and puts them all to bed in empty drawers. She slams them to sleep.

At 8:00 P.M., the nourishment cart arrives. Treats appear that help residents sleep a little longer, that keep the memory of food alive a few seconds more so they won't wander the halls at night, hungry for corn flakes too soon. Ritz crackers, Lorna Doones, slices of processed American cheese, cans of Ensure are placed in hands. Their favorite foods are served. My mother refuses to eat tonight. There isn't time.

At 8:30 P.M., people begin to slow down. Women find afghans and blankets and snuggle up in chairs. Some remember negligees and robes and flip-flop slippers in pink and powder blue and wander to their rooms to find them. Yawns are heard frequently, in every pitch, yawns written for soprano and glass harp.

At 8:45 P.M., my mother finally is ready to stop. She sits in a chair. Within ten seconds her eyes close. Her neck relaxes and spills her head forward. She is sound asleep.

Throughout the summer I watched the mute swans, and they watched me. At first I would take field guides to compare their markings and habits with the perfect pictures of Roger Tory Peterson. I found myself screeching to a stop in front of libraries and piling large reference books about swans in the back seat of my car.

The birds became an obsession. All summer, I sat on the banks of the pond and watched the swans.

Mute swans are spectacular creatures. They are the heaviest of all flying birds. They are beautiful in the air but frequently kill themselves by colliding with overhead power cables. It is the principal cause of death in swans.

Mutes can be more aggressive than other swans and have been known to kill rival mutes and predators such as dogs by pushing the other's head under water and drowning it. They have broken the legs of human beings with the force of their jointed wings. Not far into the summer, I noticed that Tanglewood's swans had driven the other waterfowl away. No geese, no ducks dared return to the pond.

Sometimes the skulls of cygnet mutes are deformed. This deformity occurs in families and is thought to be hereditary. Sometimes they die of metal poisoning: copper and zinc have been found in their alimentary tracts.

Not so long ago in Britain, the King's Swanmaster each year ordered swanherders to cut marks on the bills of cygnets, marks identical to those on the bills of their parents.

Nearly 85 percent of all mute swans stay together for life.

Long Island introduced mutes to give the lakes style and beauty. America's native swans are the trumpeter and the whistler.

Mutes can quickly be identified from other varieties

by the graceful S-shape of their necks. Other swans hold their necks severely straight, their bills perfectly horizontal. But not these birds. As you watch them work their magical necks, mutes seem to be signing. "P" appears as they preen the middle of their necks. A "D" forms as they push their bills into their chests. "M's" and "W's" line the sky when their bills touch and their necks interlock. "Z's" materialize when the S-shape is reversed and the birds rest their bellies to the ground. When they rise from this position, a giant question mark heaves in feathered mystery from the earth.

And sometimes the mute communicates in sounds, in spite of its name. Although a mute has a weaker voice than native swans, it does occasionally speak. It snorts when it's angry, and when it's excited. It hisses when frightened. When it calls its young you might mistake it for the family dog.

And sometimes—not often, but sometimes—it emits a glorious sound, like a French horn crying to be heard above all the other instruments.

CHAPTER THIRTEEN

༒

Surprises

"Don't forget, I'm inside this thing," he said, and it turned out he was right.

IAN FRAZIER, *Family*

·1·

Gloria is on the patio when her weak eyes locate the head of a mushroom in a moist corner of the garden, a corner cooled by bushes and kept wet by the trickle of a clogged downspout.

"Mushrooms!" she screams. She wobbles over to the plant and stares it down. She picks it and carries it inside.

"What do you have there?" asks a man delivering food from the central kitchen.

"Mushrooms!" she says again, even more delighted than before. Now she has an audience and can tell her story.

Gloria carries a small tapestry purse with a jeweled clasp. In it is a collection of scraps of paper, of prayers and short poems that she's composed. She finds a white slip with brown ink. On it is her poem called "Mushrooms":

> A mushroom blooms
> When twilight glooms.
> (To Be Cont'd)

She shows it to the man dressed in hospital green. "I have a picture I had made *this* big," she says, using her hands to sketch a large frame in the air. "Of mushrooms!" she whispers, proudly.

"I know," the man responds. "And you had mushroom wallpaper, mushroom clocks, and mushroom dishes. You had mushroom everything, Gloria. Your daddy harvested mushrooms."

"How do you know all that?" Gloria asks, amazed.

"I'm your nephew," he reminds her.

Gloria seems not to have heard his last words, but only the words about the mushrooms. "Dad used to come home with a whole half bushel."

Gloria gradually forgets the mushrooms too. "How do I get to the street, young man?" she asks this stranger, her nephew. "I live off Grant Street. Mother and Father have lived there since they've been married."

Her nephew smiles and helps her to a chair. Gloria seems confused. "I want Grant and Ivy. No one seems to know where it is and I've lived there all my life."

The man straightens his aunt's collar. Gloria's good cheer returns.

"Remember!" she shouts. "A week from Friday is peacocks!"

· 2 ·

I immediately spot Benny as I enter, all ninety pounds of him, slouched down in a chair in the row of rockers, grinning. I have to look twice to make sure it's really him. Dressed in a black vinyl vest, gray sweats, and tan tennis shoes, Benny is wearing sunglasses today.

It's the last week of August, the summer Saturday beach party at Tanglewood. Everyone, except my mother, knows something is about to happen. They are all sitting in the two rows of chairs in the living area, facing one another, waiting. Children's sunglasses with fluorescent rims are being passed around in a McDonald's Happy Meals bucket. Several people put them on.

A tape is inserted in the deck. Beach sounds. Water crashing on rocks, sea gulls screeching high overhead, pebbles grating on the beach as the tide comes in, goes out. Every few minutes, a ship blows a foghorn in the background, signaling distress.

"What's that noise?" Faye asks me.

"It's the ocean," I tell her.

"I thought so," Faye says. "I thought that's what it was."

The nurse and Angie unpack boxes full of beach toys and artifacts. First, a teal swimming pool is placed between the two rows of chairs. Each resident is offered a toy to throw into the rubber pool. Beanbag fish, fluffy whales and seals and dolphins and sharks. Even a Skimee, a sort of bathing pool Frisbee, appears. Other inflatable rubber toys are blown up by the aides, amazing residents.

"Throw the fish into the water," they are told. People hold fish by tails and try to remember how to position their arms for the toss.

Gloria falls in love with her gray dolphin. She approaches the nurse's station and asks if she can buy it. Maggy assures her they will order her one, and that there will be no cost. For her, it's free. She is satisfied and returns to the beach.

Fish are collected and repackaged. Then Maggy fills a larger bucket with real seashells, five inches wide, and slowly distributes them to the people who haven't yet left the party, haven't yet wandered off. She invites them to remember the feel and the shape of shells, to head for Florida or California with her. Holding the shells between her fingertips, she delicately places them in palms. "A shell from the seashore," she says in a sacred whisper, smiling. Over and over, clear around the room, "A shell from the seashore." "A shell from the seashore."

Some residents are lost, turning the shells at odd angles to examine them or testing them with their teeth for possible consumption. But a few lift them to their ears and listen.

Crackers with cream cheese and salami begin to appear on paper plates. Next, cups of lemonade. People who have wandered off drift back for this and sit.

And then, two bottles of suntan lotion suddenly float into the room. On arms and wrists are rubbed lotions of pungent oils and thick perfumes. "Smell," Maggy tells her guests, lifting limbs close to noses. They do.

From the hallway, my mother watches, a ship lost at sea. Maggy spots her and carries the orange bottle of suntan lotion toward her. Maggy places lotion on her own index finger and calms my mother until Annabelle lets her rub the ridge of her upper lip with sweet beach memories. I wonder why the nurse is doing this. My mother lost her sense of smell to her disease years ago.

Annabelle soon resists, and turns away. But as I follow at her side, she stops, just for a moment, and closes her eyes. Her shoulders rise, her chest heaves slowly, and she breathes in wind and salt and ocean spray for one last time.

· 3 ·

When I arrive at the end of summer, I immediately know something is different. My mother has allowed her hair to be cut at the beauty shop. But not just that. That is only a sign. Something is generally more youthful about her. She's moving quickly up and down the halls, loping in spurts. It's Friday afternoon.

"She bowled today!" Angie shouts to me. She hasn't helped set up the unit's large plastic pins for years. She hasn't known how to position her fingers in the holes of the weighted plastic ball. But today I'm told she bowled.

She sees me. "Come on!" she says. I can't believe what I've

heard. Two words together, in a sequence, in a pattern she's re-covered from some mysterious zone in the cortex of her decaying brain.

We race to the patio and she's off. Around the walk we go, three times. She puffs but continues on. It's 1928 and she's back in high school winning medals for gymnastics and rope climbing and speed.

"Slow down!" I say, laughing. "You're a ball of fire today." I shout these things in her ear, using phrases that I learned from her.

"That's for sure!" she says, probably not knowing what I've said but putting more words together than I ever thought I'd hear again. She pauses only long enough to pick a purple impatiens and stick it in the cuff of her sweatshirt.

She decides to return to the unit and pulls hard on the patio door. Briefly she stops by the bingo game and eyes the ten women around the table. She almost joins them. Instead an aide offers her a piece of chocolate candy, placing it between her lips, and my mother concentrates on the taste. She pushes the candy be-tween her gums and sucks.

Again she hurries to the patio, this time sitting in a lounge chair. She puts her feet up and crosses them elegantly at the ankle. She picks up today's paper from the ground. On the back of an advertising page is the huge red headline NAME BRANDS. She tries to read the first word. "AM-A-NAM." This is the closest she will ever come to recovering her former passion for reading.

The chocolate has dissolved and the candy's center begins to disturb her. There's a hard nut in the middle, a mistake for my toothless mother. She spits the nut half through her lips and tries to stare down at it. Her eyes partially cross. I take the nut from her gently and toss it into the bushes.

"Throwed it away," she says, understanding what has just hap-pened. My eyes heat with tears and under my breath I say her words over and over like the beads of a rosary. "Come on." "That's for sure." "AM-A-NAM." "Throwed it away."

I usually visit for two hours at a time, but today I stay all after-noon. I stay for supper and into the night. I stay until the sun begins to disappear. I know this day will never return. I can have it only once.

I pull my mother from her seat for one last walk. As usual, she directs me, even though her gait is showing signs of exhaustion from the summer day. This time she drags me toward the doors at the entrance to Tanglewood. I think she wants to exit with me, to wander the halls outside her world for a little while before sleep, but I am wrong.

She recognizes the brass handles of the doors, knows their meaning, and pulls, opening one wide. Then she cups her hand over my cheek and strokes it. She moves her hand toward my shoulder and gently pushes me to the other side.

"Are you saying goodbye to me? Are you trying to get rid of me?" I laugh.

She laughs too and scratches my neck with her rough nails. She spots the purple flower in her cuff as she does this and hands it to me with the words, "Cape it."

She lets the door close slowly, lets it divide us with its thick-ness. She places her lips on the cold steel over the vertical crack between the doors. I do the same on the other side.

"Goo-bye," she says.

"Goo-bye, my love," I whisper in reply.

She turns and leaves me. I hear the soft shuffle of her slippers on the carpet and peek through the narrow panes of glass to find her, but my mother is gone. I want to catch her in amber, just a speck of her, but she has disappeared, entirely. The glass is clear, empty now.

I realize that for the first time in my life I have nowhere to go. My mother has given me up, her identical twin, her orphan child, and placed me gently on someone else's doorstep with just a flower and her touch.

So I turn the other way and head toward the street, alone, thinking of her.

AFTERWORD

My mother died on February 5, 1995. She died, as I knew she would, from her primary illness. There is only one cause of death listed by her certifying physician on her Certificate of Death from the Department of Health: "End Stage Alzheimer's Disease (Rapidly Progressive)." She was no longer able to skip away from Death and escape.

Her last months were not painful for her, but they were for me. She forgot how to be hungry. She gave it up for New Year's, I guess. It was her resolution, and never, as long as I'd known her, had she broken one. For weeks, I watched her lose weight and tighten her lips to spoons and cups and even the sweetest icings. I nearly drove myself mad dreaming of how to make her remember how good food was. I made puddings and cookies with triple the sugar in the middle of the night, bought rich morning cereals from yuppie restaurants, talked to pharmacists about highly caloric shakes (those served warm, those served cold). I hired the daughter of a nurse to help feed Annabelle on the days I could not be with her. I spent entire afternoons coaxing six ounces of fluid between her lips, experimenting with favorite cups, using eye droppers, spoons, swizzle sticks, anything. Sometimes I dipped my finger into the food on her tray and let her lick.

The nurses and staff hovered around her day and night with drinks and candied yams, tempting her, coaxing her like overly attentive waiters. But I had made the painful decision not to feed her through a belly plug, the decision I thought she would have made for herself. And there was only so much any of us could do after that.

The final few weeks of her life Annabelle lived on McDonald's milkshakes.

∽

It was snowing hard the last afternoon I spent with her. The last afternoon of her life. It was the worst storm of the winter of 1995. When I arrived, cold to the bone, I found Annabelle in bed, the sides drawn as high as they would go. She was flopping from one rail to the other in her purple sweatshirt and gray running pants. Her hair was clean and shiny, but her eyes had disappeared somewhere. Her lids hung like broken shades that let in only a mysterious slit of light at the bottom. When I lifted one lid between my fingers, I was horrified that her pupils were gone. Only a blue cloud met my glance.

I tried to settle myself down. I had never seen my mother like this before. She always had managed to find enough energy to leave her bed and dance to the living room. I hurried to the nurses' station and found Esther. Frightened, I asked her to check on Annabelle, *please,* to help her straighten her clothes, fix the diaper my mother's busy hands still tried to understand after all this time. Esther hugged me and stroked my hair and then hurried to Annabelle's side.

When Esther returned, she led me softly to my mother's room. She sensed how fragile I was. I think she would have stayed with me forever, carried me in her arms until dark. But I knew she had other things to do. So I sent her out and sat watching Annabelle Coyne all afternoon. I wanted to climb into the bed with her, hold her, but her flailing told me that she did not want me there. She had to do this thing alone.

So from a chair placed at the bottom of her bed, at her foot, I just watched. But others joined me in this vigil.

All afternoon Alzheimer's residents stopped to pay tribute, and say goodbye. They sensed something was wrong. They were walking. Annabelle was not. They were making loud sounds and screams. Annabelle was silent. So one by one, they called.

First came Rebecca, a new resident, a former military colonel in her early fifties who spoke in loud gibberish, lower teeth protruding, spoke words about family—about mamma and daddy and babies. "Oh, da BABY, da BABY. Oh, da BABY, da BABY. Oh da BABY!" She repeated her refrain over and over, holding onto the railing and staring into my mother's crib. She laughed hysterically, raised an arm, and saluted. She marched away from us.

Gloria Nevel delivered a peach smile and a grin. "She needs some sleep," Gloria said to someone, no one, before walking out.

After her came Benny, snapping his suspenders with one hand and carrying a bowling trophy with the other. He sang something that was unrecognizable but pure and clear. He looked at his trophy, placed it on my mother's nightstand, and whistled his way out the door.

Frank, another new resident, a marathon runner in his late forties whose wife divorced him after his diagnosis and whose children never visited, came to inspect my mother's untouched food tray. Normally he would have consumed everything in seconds, like a blast furnace. But today he only jogged in place.

Between these visits, nurses, aides, dieticians, supervisors, activity directors, maintenance staff entered the room. Carolyn wrapped Annabelle's bed rails with soft blankets, pinning them taut at the corners. She hugged me, over and over, her huge bosom softening my pain. She spoke seldom, but smiled and blinked her eyes quickly behind her glasses.

A floor nurse talked to me about medications. I worried that my mother was suffering. She assured me she was not—just delirious. She flew across the room when she saw my eyes redden and bent down to wrap her arm around my neck. "She's going to a better place," she whispered in my ear.

The nursing supervisor came in to explain that Alzheimer's was sedative enough for even this, a natural sedative that deadened nerve cells, all recognition. My mother would never know she was sleeping with Death this afternoon.

A maintenance man mopped slowly across the linoleum, carefully attending to the milkshake and ice cream spills I had made, his sad eyes carefully attending to me.

∾

I don't plan to recover from what I've seen over the last nine years. My friends look at me with sorrow and urge me to take a good, long vacation. They are kind, but they do not understand. Alzheimer's disease is not about recovery, either for the patient or for the family members who watch.

My dear friends have not been where I have been.

Alzheimer's disease has changed me forever. The Florida sun or a Bahamas breeze will not help me forget any of this.

And why would the daughter of a woman who forgot everything find comfort in forgetfulness?

I want to remember every moment I had with my mother, including every second of the last nine years. I want to remember her toothless grin, her screams, her growing fondness for sweets and then for nothing at all, the bouquets of uprooted flowers she picked for me from her unit's patio, the way she tried to fold her bib, the rare pats to my cheek that meant everything, her last words, her last party, her last dance. And I want to remember what I learned from aides and nurses, from volunteers and cleaning staff, from my mother's own sick friends.

I don't want to forget a single thing.

APPENDIX

In 1907 a German physician named Alois Alzheimer (pronounced ALTS-hi-mer) reported changes in the brain of a fifty-five-year-old deceased man who had experienced severe dementia for five years. The cerebral cortex contained abnormal nerve cells with tangles and clusters of dying nerve endings. He identified an organic cause for dementia, and the world began to understand for the first time that dementia was the result of a disease, a dangerous and devastating and irreversible disease. Not until the '60s would much additional work be done to further document that dementia of the Alzheimer type was not the inevitable result of aging but the result of an actual disease.

The brains of people with Alzheimer's are dying. The enzyme that produces the chemical memory messenger acetylcholine is 60 to 90 percent less prevalent in the brains of those with Alzheimer's than in healthy brains. Neurons are decaying, losing their intricate branches. Odd two-stranded tangles appear within nerve cells. Plaques, lying outside the bodies of nerve cells, become the grim garbage heaps where the tireless dictator Alzheimer deposits the helpless victims of its destruction, fragments of dead or dying neurons. Brains shrink and atrophy.

Why is this happening? Why do some brains die but those of people like Pablo Casals, Georgia O'Keeffe, Eubie Blake, Konrad Adenauer, Pablo Picasso, and Rebecca West remain perfectly tuned, perfectly complete into their nineties? Why was Annabelle Coyne not so lucky?

And if luck has no place here, what can we blame for what has happened to the Annabelle Coynes of the world? For what has happened to one out of every three families in the United States?

Many theories once taken seriously no longer are. Metals like aluminum and zinc and mercury were formerly considered culprits, but few believe this any longer. There was a time not many years ago when Alzheimer's disease was thought to be caused by a virulent virus. But viral hypotheses are not popular these days. Until fairly recently the immune system and antibodies were the vigorous focus of research. But there is not much evidence that autoantibodies are playing a role in Alzheimer's. Researchers are still exploring the relationship between nutrition and AD, but the role of diet is highly speculative.

One area of research, however, may finally be leading us out of the dark night of this disease. That area is genetics.

Something is going on here. Clearly, and painfully, close relatives are at higher risk. In both "early-onset" Alzheimer's (acquired between forty and fifty) and "late-onset" Alzheimer's, children of parents with Alzheimer's are more likely to develop the disease than the general population.

Two recent studies indicate the promise of genetic research. In a winter 1996 issue of the *Journal of the American Medical Association,* a team of researchers at the University of Kentucky published revolutionary findings about a group of nuns, the School Sisters of Notre Dame. The investigators had expected to find that education and an active mind better fortified people against dementia. As a matter of fact, this expectation was announced to the American public on August 5, 1994, on an ABC *Nightline* show called "Beating Alzheimer's: The Nuns' Gift." But less than two years after that announcement, the research team, led by David Snowdon, modified their thesis that education offered protection from Alzheimer's. They would propose, instead, that nuns in their study group who would acquire the disease were perhaps developing plaques in their brains even in their twenties.

How did this radical and profound shift towards genetics occur? Four years after the ninety-three nuns in the study group (all born before 1917 and now in their eighties) entered the convent, and just before they took their vows, they were required to write brief autobiographical essays. In 90 percent of the cases, Kentucky researchers found that those nuns who went on to develop Alzheimer's disease had produced very simple prose with few complex grammatical constructions; those who escaped dementia had written autobiographies full of complex language and ideas. Autopsies on fourteen of the nuns who had died showed five brains diseased by Alzheimer's, and all five women had exhibited low idea density in their early writing. Last year a German autopsy study showed Alzheimer's plaques in people in their twenties, providing both precedent and support to the findings of David Snowdon, epidemiologist at the University of Kentucky and the lead author in the study.

Snowdon of course admits that we do not yet know exactly *why* low early linguistic ability is a predictor of the disease. It may be that high linguistic ability provides resistance to the disease. But even more likely, it may be that the disease is already fermenting when people are very young. The genetic trigger has been pulled.

A second exciting moment in Alzheimer's research occurred in 1995 when a research team led by Peter St. George-Hyslop discovered a gene linked to early-onset Alzheimer's called FAD3. Prior to this discovery—a discovery announced in the June 29, 1995, issue of *Nature*—Chromosome 21 had long been suspected by researchers of setting AD in motion. It was a logical and intelligent guess, for every person with Down's syndrome who enters middle age develops Alzheimer's disease. And every person with Down's syndrome is the carrier of a mutant form of Chromosome 21. But researchers began to find that many family groups that participated in Alzheimer's research showed no such mutations in this particular gene. As a matter of fact, 97 percent demonstrated no amyloid gene mutations.

But Peter St. George-Hyslop of the University of Toronto discovered a gene that was linked to up to 90 percent of early-onset cases. The gene is located near one end of Chromosome 14. St. George-Hyslop and his team spent years finding its exact location and extracting it from the chromosome. The team examined two hundred healthy elderly people, for even one healthy person carrying the gene would destroy St. George-Hyslop's hypothesis. But they never found it among the well.

Researchers are now trying to determine how FAD3 causes Alzheimer's symptoms. We know that it does order brain cells to make a protein that contributes to AD. But it does not seem to increase beta-amyloid production.

These advances in understanding may offer those of us born at a later time a treatment not available to our parents. At this time of writing it strongly appears that genetics will answer the difficult questions that remain. Some genetic researchers are so hopeful that they have predicted that in five years prototype drugs will be available; in ten, there may be understanding and preventative treatment; in twenty, the disease may be rare, with an onset age of eighty or eighty-five.

The research community, like every other community associated with Alzheimer's disease—nurses and doctors, writers, daughters and sons—is spending difficult and sleepless nights trying to find a way to bring our mothers, our fathers, back to us. But we cannot yet know precisely when this will happen or how it will occur. There will be many more surprises, and probably many more disappointments, before the dark night passes.

Every effort of every community is nonetheless a small victory. We must remember that. And the hundreds and thousands and millions of small victories that are ours will one day defeat this ravaging disease, and make of it only a memory.

SELECTED BIBLIOGRAPHY

Popular Handbooks and References about Alzheimer's

Aronson, Miriam K., ed. *Understanding Alzheimer's Disease.*
New York: Scribner's, 1988. A collection of essays on
pertinent topics, including early-onset Alzheimer's, genetics,
emergency situations, services, and placement. Marion
Roach has a short essay in the volume entitled "The Often
Misunderstood Younger Alzheimer Victim: A Personal
Perspective."

Beckelman, Laurie. *The Facts about Alzheimer's Disease.* New
York: Crestwood House, 1990. Using in part her experience
with her grandmother, Beckelman describes the disease, its
progression, and its causes and effects. A very simple book
but good preliminary information for the general reader.

Berg, J. M., H. Karlinsky, and A. J. Holland, eds. *Alzheimer
Disease, Down Syndrome, and their Relationship.* New York:
Oxford University Press, 1993. A collection of essays that
discuss the associations between Down's syndrome and
Alzheimer's disease. The book is perhaps most valuable to
health care professionals and researchers because of its very
technical nature.

Binstock, Robert H., Stephen G. Post, and Peter J. Whitehouse,
eds. *Dementia and Aging: Ethics, Values, and Policy Choices.*
Baltimore: The Johns Hopkins University Press, 1992. This
book examines the important conviction that it is time to
struggle actively with the ethical, moral, and policy dilemmas
posed by dementia. Articles on euthanasia, for example,
show the special difficulties of that decision for people with
AD, the difficulty of arguments that center on autonomy,
mercy, and justice.

Carroll, David L. *When Your Loved One Has Alzheimer's: A Caregiver's Guide*. New York: Harper & Row, 1989. Discusses topics pertinent to families of people with Alzheimer's disease. In addition to a review of stages in the disease and possible causes, Carroll provides extensive information about a trait of the disease that seldom is mentioned at any length—violence.

Check, William A. *Alzheimer's Disease*. New York: Chelsea House Publishers, 1989. A good background book with an introduction by C. Everett Koop. Check describes the changes that occur in the brains of people with AD, speculates on causes, explains methods used for diagnosis, and reviews treatments.

Cohen, Donna, and Carl Eisdorfer. *The Loss of Self: A Family Resource for the Care of Alzheimer's Disease and Related Disorders*. New York: W. W. Norton & Company, 1986. This book includes chapters that have practical value to families of people with dementia, chapters on topics such as choosing nursing homes and causes and costs.

Congress of the United States. *Losing a Million Minds: Confronting the Tragedy of Alzheimer's Disease and Other Dementias*. Washington, D.C.: U.S. Government Printing Office, 1987. A document requested by seven committees. A detailed and excellent resource book with very elaborate and technical bibliographies.

Davidson, Frena Gray. *The Alzheimer's Sourcebook for Caregivers*. Los Angeles: Lowell House, 1993. A book marked by great affection and compassion, but not clinically detailed. Good for someone new to the disease.

Frank, Julia. *Alzheimer's Disease: The Silent Epidemic*. Minneapolis: Lerner Publications Company, 1985. Weaves the story of Sarah with the clinical analysis necessary to understand what is happening to her. Good discussion of brain involvement and excellent photographs from PET scans showing the massive presence of inactive brain cells.

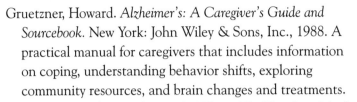

Gruetzner, Howard. *Alzheimer's: A Caregiver's Guide and Sourcebook.* New York: John Wiley & Sons, Inc., 1988. A practical manual for caregivers that includes information on coping, understanding behavior shifts, exploring community resources, and brain changes and treatments.

Heston, Leonard L., and June A. White. *The Vanishing Mind: A Practical Guide to Alzheimer's Disease and Other Dementias.* 1983 (edition called *Dementia*). New York: W. H. Freeman and Company, 1991. A very good, fairly technical account of a variety of dementias, including DAT (Dementia of the Alzheimer's Type). Provides an excellent description of tangles and plaques, information about recent therapies and treatments, and addresses of Alzheimer's-related associations.

Hodgson, Harriet. *Alzheimer's: Finding the Words.* Minneapolis: Chronimed Publishing, 1995. Provides helpful insights about dealing with one of the most profound symptoms of Alzheimer's disease—speech failure.

Mace, Nancy L., and Peter V. Rabins. *The 36-Hour Day.* 1981. Baltimore: Johns Hopkins University Press, 1991. A new edition designed to meet the special needs of families trying to cope with caring for relatives with Alzheimer's and other memory loss diseases. The first edition written in 1981 sold over half a million copies. This edition has many of the same useful chapters, but contains less jargon and includes new segments about why the demented act as they do, how to cope with angry and violent responses in the demented, "gadgets" that can be purchased to make home care easier, and new developments in nursing options.

Nuland, Sherwin B. *How We Die: Reflections on Life's Final Chapter.* New York: Alfred A. Knopf, 1994. Nuland uses a case study to show the progression of the disease, but intersperses the history of the disease, as well as what is known about cause and treatment. He finds Alzheimer's a degrading and horrible illness. This book is a good rehearsal of common knowledge, including discussions of concepts and terms like plaques, tangles, amyloids, and acetylcholine, and the prose is superior and moving.

Oliver, Rose, and Frances A. Bock. *Coping with Alzheimer's: A Caregiver's Emotional Survival Guide.* New York: Dodd, Mead & Company, 1987. A supportive text, with the focus of support on RET (Rational Emotive Therapy). Advice about anxiety, guilt, depression, and stress is given; often questions from caregivers are interspersed, and the authors answer as therapists.

Post, Stephen G. *The Moral Challenge of Alzheimer Disease.* Baltimore: Johns Hopkins University Press, 1995. In a culture that values memory and rationalism, Post argues, people with Alzheimer's disease are abandoned and denied moral, social, and political protection and rights. Human beings, he proposes, are more than powerful minds and must be treated with dignity and equality even when severely affected by dementia.

Powell, Lenore, and Katie Courtice. *Alzheimer's Disease: A Guide for Families.* Reading, Mass.: Addison-Wesley Publishing Company, 1983. Discusses symptoms, behavioral changes, and diagnostic procedures. The book emphasizes the need for support and comfort.

Reisberg, Barry. *A Guide to Alzheimer's Disease: For Families, Spouses, and Friends.* New York: Free Press, 1981. A somewhat technical, though excellent, introduction to the essentials of Alzheimer's—such topics as its origins and its treatment. Reisberg includes numerous tables and illustrations, though some are heavily detailed and may be difficult for the general reader. He also includes extensive notes after each chapter.

Sheridan, Carmel. *Failure-Free Activities for the Alzheimer's Patient.* New York: Dell Publishing, 1995. Describes activities that can generally bring satisfaction to people with Alzheimer's. Some of these include lacing, reminiscences, indoor vegetable gardening, exercising to music, and memory boxes.

Wolf-Klein, Dr. Gisèle P., and Dr. Arnold P. Levy. *Keys to Understanding Alzheimer's Disease*. New York: Barron's Educational Series, 1991. Numerous segments are offered, providing explanations and answers concerning issues key to Alzheimer's. Especially good are the discussions of stages of the disease, medical treatments, and "Sleep and Circadian Rhythms."

Adult Novels and Memoirs about Alzheimer's

Bernlef, J. *Out of Mind*. Trans. by Adrienne Dixon. Boston: David R. Godine, 1989. Written by one of the Netherlands' most celebrated writers, this novel records the voyage into senility of its narrator, an old man named Maarten. Like the narrator's mental processes, the narrative itself begins to unwind and become disjointed as familiarity and clarity gradually slip away from him.

Bryan, Jessica, ed. *Love Is Ageless: Stories About Alzheimer's Disease*. Oakland, Calif.: Serala Press, 1987. A collection of poems (some previously published) and stories by relatives facing the stress of caring for a person with Alzheimer's disease.

Caldwell, Marianne Dickerman. *Gone Without a Trace*. Forest Knolls, Calif.: Elder Books, 1995. Caldwell recounts the painful disappearance of her adoptive mother, Stella Mallory Dickerman, a woman with Alzheimer's. Stella Dickerman, an accomplished artist and weaver, vanished forever in the fall of 1991, two years after the onset of AD. The book provides information for both families of missing persons and families of people with AD. It gains special poignancy because of Caldwell's unique situation: her first mother abandoned her, and her second mother disappeared twice—disappeared through the transforming mechanisms of the disease, and literally vanished on September 13, 1991.

Coyle, Beverly. *In Troubled Waters*. New York: Ticknor & Fields,

1993. Told largely through the voice of Tom Glover, this fine story weaves prejudice against blacks in Florida (and the long history of Klanism in the state) with prejudice against Tom's son-in-law, a man who suffers from dementia.

Davis, Robert. *My Journey into Alzheimer's Disease.* Wheaton, Ill.: Tyndale House Publishers, Inc., 1989. A pastor of one of Miami's largest churches, Robert Davis, with the help of his wife, Betty, tells the story of the physical, emotional, and spiritual changes that accompany the journey into AD. It is an accurate and realistic account, but one buoyed by the religious faith of the author. It has become a standard reference for many physicians and caregivers, as well as theologians.

Dershowitz, Alan M. *The Advocate's Devil.* New York: Warner Books, 1994. A law school professor and Talmudic scholar suffering from Alzheimer's, Haskel Levine, serves as the mentor to this novel's protagonist.

Fisher, Carrie. *Delusions of Grandma.* New York: Simon & Schuster, 1994. Very little of this novel about Hollywood screenwriter Cora Sharpe is about Alzheimer's, but there are a few poignant scenes toward the end that concern the family's kidnapping of her stricken Grandpa Bill from a nursing home and their subsequent trip to his family home in Whitwright, Texas, on the train.

Frazier, Ian. *Family.* New York: Farrar, Straus and Giroux, 1994. Frazier eloquently traces the histories of his ancestors from the seventeenth century to the present, ending with the death from leukemia of his younger brother Fritz. There are Hudson, Ohio, and Western Reserve Academy segments, and several references to his father's Alzheimer's.

Gard, Robert E. *Beyond the Thin Line.* Madison: Prairie Oak Press, 1992. Gard writes about his Alzheimer's friend Harry McDare (really John Whitmore), spending considerable time imagining what goes on in Harry's mind the Christmas Eve he escapes from a nursing home.

Goldman, Abe. (with Drollene P. Brown). *Holding on to Ettie.* Plantation, Fla.: Distinctive Publishing Corp., 1991. Though the names are changed, this is essentially the story of Abe Goldman and his wife, Gertrude Neimark Goldman. The narrator is transformed by having to care for his ailing wife.

Holland, Gail Bernice. *For Sasha, with Love: An Alzheimer's Crusade.* (The Anne Bashkiroff Story.) New York: Dembner Books, 1985. Told by the author in the voice of Anne Bashkiroff. A book that deals with some of the most brutal realities of the disease and yet ends positively, describing the formation of the Family Survival Project. The project, under Anne Bashkiroff's leadership, obtained the first state-wide law in the country to help brain-damaged adults and their families.

Ignatieff, Michael. *Scar Tissue.* New York: Farrar, Straus and Giroux, 1994. A novel that tells the story of a philosophy professor from the Midwest who watches—and tries to understand—his mother's decline from Alzheimer's. In the process, he makes contact with his estranged brother, a neurologist.

King, Stephen. *Insomnia.* New York: Viking, 1994. Contains a sympathetic episode involving a once-brilliant history teacher who has lost his battle to the ravages of Alzheimer's.

McGowin, Diana Friel. *Living in the Labyrinth.* New York: Delacorte Press, 1993. This is the story of early-onset Alzheimer's, a rare account told by an AD sufferer herself. The fear, the defenses, the visits to doctors, the difficulty of an early retirement (she was a legal secretary) are all here.

Mojtabai, A. G. *Called Out.* New York: Doubleday, 1994. An air crash in Bounds, Texas, is recorded and lived through by numerous people in the town, specifically a journalist (traveling through), a waitress, a woman who owns the field where the crash occurs, a priest who gives extreme unction (now called anointing) to all victims, a man who speaks only to dogs and is the town outcast. A man with Alzheimer's, a

German Jew, is a survivor and becomes an important minor character in the novel.

Naughtin, Gerry, and Terry Laidler. *When I Grow Too Old to Dream: Coping with Alzheimer's Disease.* Australia: Collins Dove, 1991. Some background information about the disease is provided, with stories of coping and confronting the illness by caregivers (and those with AD).

Pollen, Daniel A. *Hannah's Heirs.* New York: Oxford University Press, 1993. Neurologist Dr. Daniel Pollen traces the contributions of a courageous family with familial Alzheimer's. He calls familial Alzheimer's a "personal biological Holocaust."

Roach, Marion. *Another Name for Madness: The Dramatic Story of a Family's Struggle with Alzheimer's Disease.* Boston: Houghton Mifflin Company, 1985. Records the severe difficulties the first-person narrator (and younger daughter) has coming to terms with her young mother's Alzheimer's.

Sacks, Oliver. *The Man Who Mistook His Wife for a Hat.* New York: Harper & Row, 1987. Sacks, Professor of Clinical Neurology at Albert Einstein College of Medicine, tells the stories of people suffering from neurological disorders, including Tourette's syndrome, autism, and dementia. Sacks not only describes dementia—its forms and peculiarities— but registers sympathy and admiration for sufferers who try, against all odds, to adapt and recover identity and human dignity.

Shanks, Lela Knox. *Your Name Is Hughes Hannibal Shanks: A Caregiver's Guide to Alzheimer's.* Lincoln: University of Nebraska Press, 1996. A new book with a poignant and helpful format and perspective.

Sheridan, Carmel. *Reminiscence: Uncovering a Lifetime of Memories.* San Francisco: Elder Press, 1991. Discusses a variety of ways to help older adults remember, and the importance of remembering—especially for people with dementia. Sheridan talks about life writing, games, music,

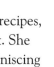

outings, photo albums, radio, TV and slides, reading, recipes, and other techniques for breaking through to the past. She argues strongly for this approach, believing that "reminiscing together gives older people a sense of their historical influence and their legacy to society, solidifying their sense of importance and accomplishment."

Shiplett, June Lund. *A Glass Full of Tears: Dementia Day-By-Day.* Cleveland: Writer's World Press, 1996. Chronicles her husband's struggle with multi-infarct dementia, an illness that in many ways resembles Alzheimer's and makes similar demands of caregivers.

Spohr, Betty Baker (with Jean Valens Bullard). *Catch a Falling Star.* Seattle: Storm Peak Press, 1995. A practical, humorous, and loving account of Betty Spohr's ten years as caregiver to her husband, Frank. The book is based on her personal journals and is cleverly illustrated with cartoon drawings.

Turner, George. *The Destiny Makers.* New York: William Morrow and Company, 1993. A science fiction novel about the premier of Australia in 2069 who is faced with a difficult decision and orders an operation on his father to reverse aging and Alzheimer's so that he can advise his son.

Adolescent Novels about Alzheimer's

Graber, Richard. *Doc.* New York: Harper & Row, 1986. Bradley Bloodworth, the narrator, has great difficulty facing the truth about his grandfather.

Kehret, Peg. *Night of Fear.* New York: Dutton, 1994. T. J. and Grandma Ruth, who has Alzheimer's, are left alone while his folks attend a school meeting. T. J. is kidnapped, but the memory of his grandmother's lessons helps him escape.

Kelley, Barbara. *Harpo's Horrible Secret.* Redfield, Ark.: Ozark Publishing, Inc., 1993. Harpo, an extremely imaginative boy, must share a room with his great-grandfather Blake. Harpo quickly puts the description of Grandpa Blake's disease

together with his own peculiar behaviors and draws the
conclusion that he, too, has Alzheimer's.

Klein, Norma. *Going Backwards*. New York: Scholastic, 1986.
An adolescent novel about a Jewish family coping with the
progressive illness of Charles Goldberg's grandmother Gustel.

Smith, Doris Buchanan. *Remember the Red-Shouldered Hawk*.
New York: G. P. Putnam's Sons, 1994. John-too welcomes his
Nanny to his house. She is extremely forgetful but still capable
of valiant acts, including turning a hose on the Ku Klux Klan.

Children's Books about Alzheimer's

Bahr, Mary. *The Memory Box*. Illus. by David Cunningham.
Morton Grove, Ill.: A. Whitman, 1992. Tells the story of
Zach's vacation on the lake his grandparents own and his
realization that his Gramps is sick with Alzheimer's. They
remember their times together for the rest of the vacation
and put their memories in the Memory Box.

Guthrie, Donna. *Grandpa Doesn't Know It's Me*. Illus. by Katy
Keck Arnsteen. New York: Human Sciences Press, 1986. Told
from the point of view of Lizzie, the book records Grandpa's
gradual decline from independent living to day care.

Karkowsky, Nancy. *Grandma's Soup*. Illus. by Shelly Haas.
Rockville, Md.: Kar-Ben Copies Inc., 1989. A young girl
named Eve, and her family, begin to notice Grandma's
confusion when she puts cloves or too much pepper in the
soup she makes for Shabbat.

Kibbey, Marsha. *My Grammy*. Illus. by Karen Ritz. Minneapolis:
Carolrhoda Books, 1988. Grammy moves in with her
daughter and shares a room with her granddaughter—the
narrator of the story. The granddaughter resents and fears
her at first, but ends up feeling very close to her.

Potaracke, Rochelle. *Nanny's Special Gift*. Illus. by Mark
Mitchell. New York: Paulist Press, 1993. Seven-year-old
Patrick persuades his family to have a picnic with blackberry

pie and mint tea at Nanny's new "home"—"Heart 'N Home"—with Nanny's friends.

Sanford, Doris. *Maria's Grandma Gets Mixed Up.* Illus. by Gracia Evans. Portland: Multnomah, 1989. Maria, a Mexican girl, is confused by her grandma's behavior, and prays to God to help her understand her grandma and to heal her. At the end, the child vows love and allegiance, "no matter what."

Schein, Jonah. *Forget-me-not.* Illus. by Jonah Schein. Toronto: Annick Press, 1988. Written by a nineteen-year-old to help explain the emotions children feel in the presence of relatives with Alzheimer's.

Whitelaw, Nancy. *A Beautiful Pearl.* Illus. by Judith Friedman. Morton Grove, Ill.: A. Whitman, 1991. Since she was born, Lisa's grandmother has given her a pearl every birthday for a necklace that will be complete when she is grown. But Alzheimer's has gotten in the way of normal habits, and Lisa fears there will be no more beads.

Poetry about Alzheimer's

Malyon, Carol. *Emma's Dead.* Toronto: Wolsak and Wynn, 1992. A very fine collection of poems about Emma, a woman Malyon claims is a figment of her imagination. It begins with Emma's death and works back to her birth—a curious reversal that is both strange and dramatic.

Morgan, Betty. *Alzheimer's Alters Us All.* Lexington: Betty Morgan, 1984. Morgan's poems deal with the stresses on the caregiver as well as the changes in people suffering from dementia.

Short Stories about Alzheimer's

Dorner, Marjorie. "Before the Forgetting." *Winter Roads, Summer Fields.* Minneapolis: Milkweed Editions, 1992. In her first volume of literary fiction, Dorner creates a fictive community called Hammern Township (with map) and supplies genealogies of major families. This, the last story, is told from the point of view of a ninety-four-year-old woman with AD, Katherine Schroeder Braegger.

Watanabe, Sylvia. "Anchorage." *Talking to the Dead.* New York: Doubleday, 1992. Little Grandma takes care of the narrator's father, Koshiro, but his behavior is worsening. Little Grandma's daughter Aunt Pearlie wants her to admit him to a home. This issue is the focus of the story. At the end, through an event both comic and sad, even Little Grandma sees that the disease is taking her son from her and that she must give him up.

Plays about Alzheimer's

Carson, Jo. *Daytrips.* New York: Dramatists Play Service, 1991. This is a memory play, ironically. Times mix and bleed into one another, as do transformations in ages of characters: only three characters appear, but two play double parts. We see Ree/Irene caught in typical Alzheimer's behaviors—being lost, not being able to go to the bathroom without help, thinking her husband is taking orders from another man about not letting her drive. The play raises the issue of whether murder or suicide might not be better options than this disease.

Essays about Alzheimer's

Collins, Glenn. "Enduring a Disease That Steals the Soul." *New York Times,* 10 November 1994, sec. C, p. 8. Reflecting on the illness of his father, Glenn concludes that AD is the cruelest and most unpredictable of all diseases. He places his discussion within the framework of Ronald Reagan's illness.

Dyer, Daniel. "Why Is Alzheimer's Funny?" *Cleveland Plain Dealer,* 24 January 1995, sec. B, p. 11. Based on his personal experience with his mother-in-law, Annabelle Coyne, Dyer

discusses the insensitivity of the national media to
Alzheimer's disease.

Gordon, Mary. "My Mother Is Speaking from the Desert."
New York Times Magazine, 19 March 1995, sec. 6, pp. 44+.
Gordon deals with the details—both physical and
emotional—that accompany the care of her elderly mother, a
complicated woman suffering from dysphoria and depression,
as well as senile dementia. Gordon deals, especially, with the
implications of memory loss on parents and children.
Her writing is eloquent, lyrical, and powerfully realistic.

Henig, Robin Marantz. "Is Misplacing Your Glasses
Alzheimer's?" *New York Times Magazine,* 24 April 1994, sec.
6, pp. 72–76. A brief background to the disease for general
readers. Henig is careful to point out that other diseases—
depression, thyroid imbalance, vitamin B-12 deficiency—
often look like AD, but are treatable. He provides a
respectable overview of the disease, along with many
common statistics.

St. George-Hyslop, P. H., et. al. "Cloning of a Gene Bearing
Missense Mutations in Early-Onset Familial Alzheimer's
Disease." *Nature* 375 (1995): 754–60. A team of researchers
led by St. George-Hyslop reports the discovery of a gene
(FAD3) linked to 90 percent of familial Alzheimer's
cases.

Snowdon, David, et. al. "Linguistic Ability in Early Life and
Cognitive Function and Alzheimer's Disease in Late Life."
Journal of the American Medical Association 279 (1996):
528–32. A description of his work with the sisters of Notre
Dame, revealing the thesis that analysis of early writing is a
strong predictor of AD.

Thomas, Lewis. "The Problem of Dementia." *Late Night Thoughts
on Listening to Mahler's Ninth Symphony.* New York: The
Viking Press, 1983. Thomas calls Alzheimer's a "disease-of-
the-century," the "worst of all diseases." He pleads for money

from government and private corporations to build a ten-year or longer foundation of research into senile dementia.

Songs/Albums about Alzheimer's

Long, Herral. *Memories of Love*. Released October 16, 1995, by Herral Long. Contact composer at the *Toledo Blade,* Toledo, Ohio.

Cartoons/Comics about Alzheimer's

Batiuck and Ayers. *Crankshaft*. November 1995. Mediagraphics, Inc. Distributed by Universal Press Syndicate.

Art Exhibits about Alzheimer's

"Willem de Kooning: The Late Paintings, the 1980s." The San Francisco Museum of Modern Art. 1996. Also on tour in Minneapolis, New York, Germany, and Holland. This exhibit of de Kooning's paintings from 1980 to 1987 documents his creative process in the face of dementia and gives a visual representation of Alzheimer's itself. The artist was diagnosed with Alzheimer's in 1989, when de Kooning was eighty-five.

Videos/Movies/Television Programs about Alzheimer's

Alzheimer's Disease. Produced and distributed by Films for the Humanities and Sciences. 1994–95. An adaptation of a Phil Donahue program that focuses on the devastating effects of Alzheimer's disease on both AD-affected individuals and family members.

Alzheimer's Disease. Produced by KERA-TV and distributed by PBS Video/Public Broadcasting Service. Life Matters Series. 1988. Depicts the daily difficulties and routines of Lee and Mary Rose as they struggle together to try to cope with Lee's Alzheimer's disease.

Alzheimer's Disease—A Daughter's Perspective. Produced by Art

Dell Orto and distributed by Boston University. 1986. Discloses the effects on family members of having an Alzheimer's disease relative, concentrating on a daughter's response to the changes in her father.

Alzheimer's Disease—A Family Perspective. Produced and distributed by Good Samaritan Hospital Department of Medical Education. Looks with care and sensitivity at the ways family members communicate with relatives who have Alzheimer's disease. The video refuses to shy away from difficult topics.

Alzheimer's Disease. Larry King Live. CNN. Broadcast June 6, 1996, 9:00 P.M. An emotional panel discussion about Alzheimer's with Angie Dickinson, Shelley Fabares, Tim Ryan, and Senator Jay Rockefeller, well-known celebrities who have witnessed the ravages of the disease on parents, siblings, and spouses. Larry King and his guests are also joined by Dr. Zaven Khachaturian, a physician with the Ronald and Nancy Reagan Research Institute.

Alzheimer's Disease: The Long Nightmare. Produced and distributed by Films for the Humanities and Sciences. 1994–95. An informative video that looks at not only the emotional problems of caring for people with Alzheimer's, but also at financial issues, recent research, and care options.

Alzheimer's Disease—Pieces of the Puzzle. Produced and distributed by University of Arizona. A set of five videocassettes that covers a wide range of topics pertinent to Alzheimer's disease and other forms of dementia. Approaches to caring for Alzheimer's-affected individuals are the concentration of the series, with advice and ideas about recreational activities, aberrant behaviors, and communication techniques.

Alzheimer's Disease Series. Produced by Hospital Satellite Network and distributed by Amer Journal of Nursing. 1985. A film designed especially for nurses, but helpful to family caregivers as well who are looking for ways to identify particular stresses and problems of the disease and means for intervention.

Alzheimer's Disease—A Son's Perspective. Produced by Art Dell Orto and distributed by Boston University. 1986. Concentrates on issues of seeking support and custodial care for people with AD, focusing on a son's role and involvement.

Alzheimer's Disease—Stolen Tomorrows. Produced by Lincoln General Hospital Education and Staff Development and distributed by Aims Media Inc. 1986. Introduces viewers to information about Alzheimer's disease and to essential strategies for successful coping.

Alzheimer's: Effects on Patients and Their Families. Produced and distributed by Films for the Humanities and Sciences. 1994–95. A study of the effects of Alzheimer's on family members, but also a close and informative look at what we know about the disease (including its response to drugs and other strategies) and what we have yet to learn.

An Alzheimer's Story. Produced by Kenneth Paul Rosenberg, M.D., and Ruth Neuwald. Distributed by Filmakers Library. 1986. Follows a woman who suffers from AD, Anna Jasper, for two years. We see dramatic changes in Anna and watch the struggle of her daughter, Zena, and her husband, Jack, as they deal with these changes. We feel the burden and pain of decisions that must be made, such as placement of Anna in a long-term nursing facility.

"Beating Alzheimer's: The Nun's Gift." *Nightline.* ABC. Broadcast August 5, 1994. Explores the possible role of early education and nutrition in the ability to resist Alzheimer's through observing and interviewing the School Sisters of Notre Dame, a group of elderly nuns who have permitted researchers to autopsy their brains at death.

Complaints of a Dutiful Daughter. Written and directed by Deborah Hoffmann. Available from Women Make Movies, 462 Broadway, Suite 500C, New York, NY 10013. Or call

(212) 925-0606 or fax (212) 925-2052. A superior and
artistic documentary produced by Deborah Hoffmann about
her mother, Doris Hoffmann. The filmmaker breaks many
taboos surrounding the disease, including the prohibition
that there is nothing comic about Alzheimer's disease.
Hoffmann focuses on milestones of the disease—The Dentist
Period, The Hearing Aid Period, The Lorna Doone Period,
The Podiatrist Period, The Ticket Period, The Social Security
Period, The Banana Period, and The Suitcase Period. She
also talks about the importance of finding a care facility
exclusively for Alzheimer's residents, a facility where people
understand and accept dementia as the norm.

"Forget Me Never." *Prime Time.* ABC. A fifteen-minute account
of the story of Diana McGowin, a woman with early-onset
Alzheimer's who chronicled her story in her book, *Living in
the Labyrinth.*

"The Long Goodbye." *CNN Presents.* Broadcast February 18,
1996, 9:00 P.M. A one-hour personal account that weaves
the story of one man who has Alzheimer's, Cary Henderson,
with commentary by Bruce Morton and interviews with Jay
Rockefeller, Dr. Daniel Pollen, Keith Hernandez, Mike Myers,
Shelley Fabares, Angie Dickinson, the Sisters of Notre Dame,
residents and owners of an Alzheimer's unit in California, and
members of a support group at Duke University. An excellent
look at the scope and painful dimension of AD, as well as at
the most recent theory and research about the illness.

Mystery of Memory. Produced by WGBH Educational
Foundation and distributed by MTI Film & Video. 1989.
Explores the relationship between memory loss and aging,
also examining the role of environment.

The Silent Epidemic. Produced by Granada Television
International and distributed by Filmakers Library. 1982.
Outlines the symptoms of the disease and discusses the
extraordinary and unique problems of caring for people
with AD.

There Were Times, Dear. Produced by Lilac Productions and distributed by Direct Cinema. 1986. Follows an AD-affected individual, Bob Millard, over a period of several years.

You Must Remember This: Inside Alzheimer's Disease. Produced and directed by Helen Bowden and Susan MacKinnon. Distributed by Filmakers Library. Interweaves the stories of several AD-affected individuals and their families with commentary from professionals. The documentary provides a total picture of the disease, including the stories of people in both early and late stages.

Internet Resources about Alzheimer's

If you enter the word "Alzheimer's" in your search engine, you will find numerous web-sites you can access. Those listed below are some of the best.

Alzheimer's Association. http://www.alz.org/

Alzheimer's Disease: A Selected List of Books for the Public (Alzheimer's Association). http://www.alz.org/lib/rlists/pubbib.html

Alzheimer's Disease Education & Referral Center (National Institute on Aging). http://wwu.cais.net/adear/

Alzheimer's Family Care. http://www.alzheimers.familycare.com/

Alzheimer's Web. http://werple.mira.net.au/~dhs/ad.html

E-mail Discussion Group. majordomo@wubios.wustl.edu (Type "Subscribe Alzheimer")

Gopher Sites. gopher:/wubios.wustl.edu:70/11/alzheimer

COPYRIGHT ACKNOWLEDGMENTS

ABOUT THE AUTHOR

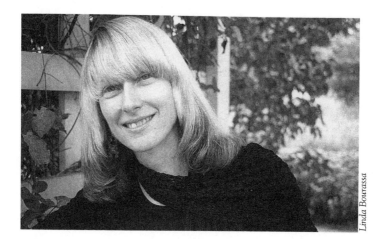

Linda Bourassa

JOYCE DYER is director of writing and associate professor
of English at Hiram College in Hiram, Ohio, where she
teaches courses in writing. She has published over a
hundred essays in journals and popular magazines. Her
first book, on author Kate Chopin, was selected by editors
of *Choice* to appear on their 1995 list of Outstanding
Academic Books. She currently is editing a collection of
reminiscences by Appalachian women writers.